Inventing Disease and Pushing Pills

Sexually unsatisfied?
Chronically tired?
Menopausal?
High cholesterol?

Don't be fooled into believing that you are sick – you are healthier than you think!

The pharmaceutical industry is redefining health, making it a state that is almost impossible to achieve. Many normal life processes – states as natural as birth, ageing, sexuality, unhappiness and death – are systematically being reinterpreted as pathological, thus creating new markets for their treatments. In this enlightening book, Jörg Blech reveals:

- how the invention of diseases by pharmaceutical companies is turning us all into patients, and how we can protect ourselves against this;
- how the medical profession has been bullied and coopted into endorsing profitable cures for people who aren't ill;
- fears about how pharmaceutical companies create markets by playing on the general public's concern with their health.

Inventing Disease and Pushing Pills is an accessible and reassuring account of how the pharmaceutical industry is eradicating health. It will appeal to doctors, nurses and all medical professionals as well as the general public.

Jörg Blech studied biology and biochemistry at the University of Cologne, Germany and the University of Sussex, UK. He then trained as a journalist and was awarded internships in Paris, Washington DC and Bangkok. He is the science correspondent for the magazine *Der Spiegel* and lives with his family in Arlington, Massachusetts.

Inventing Disease and Pushing Pills

Pharmaceutical companies and the medicalisation of normal life

Jörg Blech

Translated by Gisela Wallor Hajjar

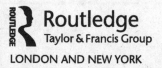

Routledge
Taylor & Francis Group

LONDON AND NEW YORK

First published in 2003 with the title *Die Krankheitserfinder*
by S. Fischer Verlag, Frankfurt

First published in the UK 2006 by Routledge
4 Park Square, Milton Park, Abingdon, Oxon OX14 4RN
605 Third Avenue, New York, NY 10017

Routledge is an imprint of the Taylor & Francis Group,
an informa business

© S. Fischer Verlag GmbH, Frankfurt am Main 2003
This English translation authorised by Fischer Verlag
Copyright © 2006 Taylor & Francis

Typeset in Sabon by BC Typesetting Ltd, Bristol BS31 1NZ

British Library Cataloguing in Publication Data
A catalogue record for this book is available from the British Library

Library of Congress Cataloging in Publication Data
A catalog record has been requested for this book

ISBN13: 978-0-415-39069-9 (hbk)
ISBN13: 978-0-415-39071-2 (pbk)

For Anke,
with love and thanks

Contents

Preface

According to Voltaire, the art of the medical profession consists in amusing the patient for as long as it takes nature to cure him or her. Nowadays, the French philosopher's wisdom is being upturned: modern medicine persuades individuals that nature scourges them with ever-new diseases – diseases which can be cured only by doctors. Because every culture creates its own ailments, disease has been considered, until recently, a social phenomenon. Here I report on how things have changed in industrial nations. Nowadays, pharmaceutical companies and medical associations are inventing diseases – illness is becoming an industrial product. In doing so, these companies and associations transform normal life processes into medical problems. They *medicalise* life.

How far this process has already progressed and how seriously it affects our society, our health system and each one of us are matters that have barely been touched upon let alone discussed in any depth. This book aims to change that. It describes the sell-out of our health and the rules that govern the process in order that we may be better equipped to shield ourselves.

The disease mongers have been overlooked until now for two reasons. In the first instance, pharmaceutical companies and physicians tirelessly claim that the public is actively seeking their help and demanding treatment. This argument is nothing but a flimsy excuse. Doubtlessly, it is part of human nature to strive for good health. However, the disease mongers nourish this desire, calculate it so that it meets their own purpose and exploit it deliberately.

In the second instance, the disease mongers have been operating behind closed doors and as a result they have been able, until now, to avoid a comprehensive account of their practices. To question my attempt, as a non-physician, to produce such an account would be the weakest kind of argument against this book. I am a natural scientist and a journalist. Tracking down facts and research findings which are not easily obtainable is my profession. I can look back upon a decade of experience as a medical editor, at first at the *Stern* and the *Zeit*, and now at the *Spiegel*. In addition to examples from German-speaking regions, I have also included Anglo-Saxon sources for evaluation, particularly since the 'fabrication and marketing' of diseases has become a global trend.

Moreover, many of the research papers and opinions that I am presenting in this book are those of physicians. Their studies and commentaries are scattered across various specialist journals and so have barely attracted public attention. It was my goal to gather knowledge about the fabrication of diseases into a book which would be quickly and comprehensively informative.

An opposing movement is also described in this book. A large and, according to my observation, growing number of medical doctors are rebelling against the medicalisation of life pursued by the pharmaceutical industry and its medical accomplices. In their eyes, the ethos of the physician is worth far more any day than the grim prospect of turning healthy people into sick ones. They dislike the creeping transformation of surgeries into sales outlets.

What I have in common with those critical physicians is that I am not turning against the pharmaceutical industry or not against modern medicine at any rate. I have my flu injections and attend cancer prevention screenings. The dilemma, however, lies in the fact that medicine has reached a stage where it is difficult to recognise the state of one's own health. This was the trigger for writing the book. I wrote it because I want to stay healthy.

Hamburg, January 2005

Acknowledgements

This book is based on the groundwork of many people to whom I owe a debt of gratitude. Exploring their knowledge and thoughts has been a pleasure; condensing them into my book was hard work.

I am especially grateful to the physicians who talked me through the medicalisation of life and provided me with invaluable suggestions. Professor Dr Peter Riedesser, psychiatrist at the University Clinic Hamburg-Eppendorf, supplied me with source material and intriguing findings that were of great benefit. Professor Dr Asmus Finzen from the University Hospital Basle took me on a tour through the world of psychiatric diagnostics. Professor Dr Hartmut Porst, Hamburg, explained about the connections between physicians and the pharmaceutical industry.

My thanks also go to Professor Dr Peter Sawicki, professor of internal medicine and partner of the German Institute for evidence-based Medicine (DIeM) in Cologne. He kindly examined the manuscript for errors and plausibility. Whatever errors remain of course are down to me.

I am particularly grateful to my friend, Jobst-Ulrich Brand, whom I met while attending the Hamburger Journalisten Schule. He read the complete manuscript and, with his feeling for language, he tamed my overly adventurous expressions and brought me closer to achieving my goal of writing a readable book.

Alfred Barthel from the Pressedatenbank Gruner + Jahr searched through an enormous amount of material and supplied me with a profusion of invaluable sources and articles. Matthias Landwehr and his colleagues at the agency Eggers & Landwehr shared my enthusiasm for the idea of this book and represented it professionally. Nina Bschorr, my editor at S. Fischer, was committed to this book and offered splendid encouragement for its production at her publishing house. The *Spiegel Verlag* generously allowed me to complete this project.

I wrote this book during holidays and at weekends. My biggest thanks go to my wife Anke Bördgen and our three children. My wife has encouraged me in this project from its inception through to the completion of the proofs; her support has made it possible to write this book. With love and tranquillity she ensured that it was written in a mood both positive and relaxed.

Translator's acknowledgements:
Special thanks to Annette L. Karseras, Sumi and Cai and Manuela and Eileen Hajjar.

1 Limitless healing

Medicine is so ahead of its time that nobody is healthy any more.
Aldous Huxley

At the beginning of the twentieth century, a doctor named Knock
started to exorcise the healthiness from his patients. The Frenchman
longed for a world which contained only patients: 'Every well person
is a sick person who doesn't know it.'

Knock put his theory into practice in a mountain village called Saint
Maurice. The residents were in good health and didn't go to the
doctor. The old country doctor, the impoverished Dr Parpalaid, tried
to console his successor and said to him: 'Here you have the best
kind of clientele ever: one is left in peace.' Knock wasn't going to
accede to this.

But how was the new doctor going to lure fit people into his surgery?
What was it that he was going to prescribe to the healthy? Knock cunningly flatters the village teacher and gets him to give the residents talks
about the alleged dangers of micro-organisms. He engages the village
drummer and induces him to announce that the new doctor invites
all residents to a free consultation – in order to 'prevent the perilous
spread of all kinds of diseases now circulating in our once so healthy
region'. The waiting room is getting crowded.

During surgery hours Knock diagnoses peculiar symptoms and
hammers into the guileless villagers that they are in need of his constant care. From then on, many stay in bed and restrict their intake
to a little water. Finally, the whole village seems to be one big hospital.
There remain just enough healthy people to look after the ill. The
pharmacist becomes a rich man; the same goes for the landlord,
whose pub, transformed into a makeshift infirmary, is fully occupied
at all times.

In the evenings, Knock delightedly glances at the ocean of lights surrounding him: the 250 brightly lit sickrooms, where – as prescribed by the doctor – 250 thermometers are inserted into the appropriate orifices, as soon as the clock strikes ten. 'And almost all the light belongs to me', Knock muses rapturously to himself. 'Those who aren't sick sleep in the darkness, they're not important.'[1]

The three-act play *Dr Knock or the Triumph of Medicine* celebrated its glittering premiere in 1923 in Paris. During the following four years, the play by the French playwright Jules Romains was staged 1,400 times and later turned into several films. It is still being performed in schools to this day. Dr Knock is irrepressible – his medicine has outlived the stage and is moving on to real life. This is the story that will be told here: it describes how healthy people are turned into patients.

Nowadays it is not a cunning doctor whose lights shine in the sickrooms. A power incomparably stronger has lined up to cure people of their health: modern medicine. Medical associations and pharmaceutical companies, often supported by patient groups, lecture us at the beginning of the new century, and proclaim an art of healing which no longer features healthy people.

To keep up the enormous growth of earlier years, the health industry is increasingly forced to stalk the healthy. Globally operating pharmaceutical firms and internationally networked medical associations are defining our health in new ways: natural vicissitudes and normal modes of behaviour are systematically being reinterpreted as pathological. Pharmaceutical companies are sponsoring the invention of a whole catalogue of clinical pictures, thus creating new markets for their products.

The firms Jenapharm and Dr Kade/Besins in Berlin are currently trying to publicise a disease which allegedly afflicts men in their prime: the 'Ageing Male Syndrome' – the male menopause. The two firms engaged opinion research institutes, public relations (PR) corporations, advertising agencies and medical professors to announce the male menopause. At press conferences, complaints were voiced about the 'insidious loss' of male hormone production. The impetus for this campaign is two hormone preparations which were launched on the German market in April 2003 (see Chapter 8).

It is within the repertoire of the disease mongers to extend the original use of a medicament. The wake-up-pill Provigil is licensed in the United States for the treatment of the rare disease narcolepsy, characterised by sudden sleeping attacks. To enlarge the circle of consumers, the manufacturer Cephalon is trying to find clinical pictures to capture the public imagination. The firm sponsored a study that found the narcolepsy tablet could help restless children. It researched the condition of shift workers – and sure enough is claiming to have discovered a new disorder 'night shift sleep disturbance'.[?]

'It is easy to create new diseases and new treatments', states the *British Medical Journal.* 'Many of life's normal processes – birth, ageing, sexuality, unhappiness and death – can be medicalised.'[3] The expansion of diagnoses in the industrial nations has reached grotesque dimensions. Physicians claim to have discovered almost 40,000 different epidemics, syndromes, disorders and diseases in Homo sapiens.

For every ill, there is a pill – and more and more often for every new pill, there is a new disease as well. In the English language, the phenomenon has already been named: 'disease mongering' – dealing in diseases. Disease mongers earn their money by persuading healthy people that they are ill. Don't you too suffer occasionally from sleepiness, a bad temper or lack of enthusiasm? Do you sometimes have trouble concentrating? Are you timid?

In the media, you will inescapably and slightly unsettlingly discover a whole range of diseases which could apply to you: high blood pressure, social phobia, jetlag, Internet addiction, elevated cholesterol level, disguised depression, obesity, menopause, fibromyalgia, irritable bowel syndrome or erectile dysfunction. Medical societies, patient groups and pharmaceutical firms are informing the public in never-ending media campaigns about disorders that are allegedly serious yet treated far too rarely.

The so-called 'Sisi-syndrome' emerged for the first time in 1998 in a one-page advertisement by SmithKline Beecham (nowadays GlaxoSmithKline). According to the firm, the affected patients were depressive and could be treated with psycho-pharmaceuticals, but by pretending to be particularly active and life affirming, these patients were glossing over their pathological depression. The syndrome was called after the Austrian Empress Elisabeth (nicknamed 'Sisi'), who was the archetype of patients suffering from the condition. This syndrome is now being propagated by some psychiatrists: in Germany some three million people are said to be suffering from Sisi-syndrome.

In May 2003, medical consultants from the University Clinic Münster exposed the popular syndrome as an invention of the industry. Their analysis of specialist literature showed that the clinical picture presented was scientifically unfounded. The media presence of Sisi-syndrome included the launch of a technical book about the subject and could be traced back to Wedopress, a PR firm in Oberursel that followed instructions from GlaxoSmithKline. Wedopress itself is boasting that in order to promote 'the introduction of a "new" depression', it had 'paved the way for "Sisi-syndrome" to hit the media'.[4]

Interestingly, the original inventor of the syndrome, a medical doctor and freelance consultant to the company, proposed to name it 'Diana-syndrome'. This idea crossed his mind while he was reading a magazine article about the life and tragic death of the Princess of Wales. According to the medical doctor, workers at SmithKline Beecham headquarters in Munich were excited by the idea of creating a new disease and associating it with a very prominent person. However, the company, which was actually British, did not want to have the disease named after Diana, evidently for reasons of reverence towards the widely worshipped princess. Thus, the 'Diana-syndrome' became the 'Sisi-syndrome'. The Austrian empress is well known in German-speaking countries through some highly popular movies and consequently the Sisi-syndrome was confined to Germany, Switzerland and Austria.

'It's clever, witty and a bit nasty to persuade people they have something they did not know existed', comments Jacques Leibowitch, doctor at the Raymond Poincaré Hospital near Paris.[5]

The disease mongers are largely profiting from the fact that the information monopoly on health education has fallen into their hands. A collaborator of the PR agency Ogilvy Healthcare, Düsseldorf, Germany, estimates that about '70 to 80 per cent' of all articles and media coverage of medical subjects are the result of well-directed PR work. Sometimes the opinion-makers use newspapers and TV stations as so-called 'media partners' to promote their campaigns. Most of the time, however, they operate only behind the scenes. Chapter 2 describes how well-prepared 'Disease Awareness Campaigns' let clinical pictures – and as a result the fear of these illnesses – seep into our daily lives.

'People living in Germany are all affected by a vitamin deficiency', announces the Society for Nutritional Medicine and Dietetics in Aachen. In the Ruhr region 'two thirds of over 45s are at high risk of cardiac infarction', reports the *Physicians Newspaper*. More than three million German citizens are suffering from chronic fatigue syndrome and rheumatism, claims Düsseldorf's *Medical Press*, but adds, 'We are not responsible for the accuracy of this information.'

Every fifth husband and father, usually reliable and patient with the children, becomes affected by the recently discovered 'caged tiger syndrome', asserts the professor for general medicine Klaus Wahle from Münster and the PR firm Medical Consulting Group. Because of specific and until now unidentified imbalances in the brain, the fathers 'were unable to make good decisions and were at odds with every-thing and everybody. Like a trapped tiger in its cage'. In such cases, psycho-pharmacon which one could re-establish 'a harmonious balance of messenger agents' in fathers' brains.

Half (51 per cent) of the population suffer from 'reflux symptoms causing a diminished quality of life', announces a general practitioner from Rödental in Bavaria, Germany. What she means is heartburn. The private Kölner Klinik Am Ring claims to have counted exactly 822,595 people in Germany with hyperhidrosis. Those affected by the condition are sweating – allegedly so strongly as to be in need of medical care.

Nobody has counted the number of goggle-eyes, hooked noses, dumbo ears and bow legs. Dr Norbert Schweizer from Tübingen, how-ever, announces: 'An unpleasant appearance can be rated in itself as a medical condition.' In Germany plastic surgeons perform, every year, an estimated 300,000 to 500,000 cosmetic operations – and as they do so, they cut each time into healthy flesh.

Pensioners in Majorca are ready for the island doctor. In spite of – or more to the point because of – the most agreeable external conditions, they are affected by 'paradise-depression'. Psychotherapist Eckhard Neumann practising in sunny Spain claims to have noticed this con-dition.[6] 'Leisure sickness', the pathological inability to enjoy leisure, seems similarly threatening. Ad Vingerhoets from the Dutch University of Tilburg suggests that three per cent of the population is getting ill through leisure. The symptoms range from tiredness, headaches and aching extremities to vomiting and depression. Holiday resorts were to be avoided, since the scourge is particularly rampant there.[7]

Those pleasure-seekers who do not succumb to the perils of sun and leisure are also doomed to fall into the clutches of medicine. Very lively people suffer, it seems, from a 'general cheerfulness disorder'. This cheerfulness syndrome, described in the journal *Forum der Psycho-analyse*, manifests itself in symptoms like carefreeness and loss of reality.[8] Even those who manage to escape medical attention might be medical cases after all: Two to three per cent of citizens are, accord-ing to the German Society for Psychiatry, Psychotherapy and Mental Health, suffering from a pathological fear of the doctor, the 'blood and medicine phobia'.

'Give back to me my youth', writes Goethe in *Faust*. Now, a new devilish pact has been made. An alliance of physicians, pharmaceutical concerns and patients nourishes the utopian ideal of a flawless human being. Healthy people swallow life-enhancing medication in an attempt to be better than well. The number of such drugs has clearly increased in recent years: remedies to improve the brain metabolism (nootropics), psycho-pharmaceuticals, hormones, vitamin A preparations or the bacterial toxin botulinum, for example, are aimed at perfecting the well-being of health-addicted consumers.

Health is being turned into a state which nobody can attain any more, but for which one has to hand over to the health services an ever-increasing share of one's salary.

Phenomenal pharmaceutical business

While increasing costs are weighing heavily on health systems, the pharmaceutical industry is doing good business. In 2001, a year of general crisis, the profits of the ten biggest pharmaceutical enterprises increased again, by a staggering 18 per cent. This wealthy arm of the industry is spending more money on marketing than on research. Major pharmaceutical companies use one-third of their profits and one-third of their personnel to place medicines on the market. In the process, diseases are exaggerated or invented.

'The marketing people always beat [hype] these things up. It's just natural enthusiasm', said Fred Nadjarian, manager of the Roche firm in Australia, to the *British Medical Journal*. At the end of the 1990s, Roche wanted to market the antidepressant Aurorix, which is supposed to help relieve social phobia, an allegedly pathological form of shyness. A press statement sponsored by Roche claimed that more than a million Australians were suffering from the 'soul-destroying' syndrome, which could be treated with behavioural therapy and medication.

In view of the vast market, Nadjarian was already gleefully rubbing his hands – but as it turned out, he and his people weren't able to gather enough test subjects for clinical studies. Social phobia was far less common than Roche employees had initially persuaded themselves, and later the public. This fiasco, Nadjarian admits, reveals a problem within the pharmaceutical industry – namely the tendency to exaggerate. 'If you added up all the statistics', says the manager, 'we all must have about 20 diseases. A lot of these things are blown out of all proportion.'[9] A number of physicians find this fad irritating. For example, Hermann Füeßl from the district hospital in Haar complains: 'Epidemiologically dubious studies exaggerate the dimensions of problems, so they reach gigantic dimensions, in order to show the affected person that he is "in good company".'[10]

Physicians, particularly consultants, attain a higher status, gain influence and earn more money when they extend the frontiers of medical science. Professors of respected universities in Germany climb into the ring – as if it were a matter of course – to be opinion-makers for the pharmaceutical industry. An average 'front and sport' (cruel mockery) pockets fees ranging between 3,000 and 4,000 Euros for a lecture or an appearance at a press conference and openly advertises the respective products for the diseases under discussion.

'If there is no disease, the drug companies are out of business', says Carlos Sonnenschein, health expert at the Boston Tufts University. 'The tragedy of science is that medical people are prepared to sell their expertise to serve the interests of the pharmaceutical companies.'[11]

For a number of pharmaceutical firms, equipment producers and physicians' groups the well-directed medicalisation of human problems lays the foundations of their business. But the media profit as well, as they tout unfounded reports to the public. 'Many journalists and editors still delight in mindless medical formulas, where fear mongering about the latest killer disease is accompanied by news about the latest wonder drug', complains the *British Medical Journal* in one of its leading articles.[12]

Most of the data regarding public health are gathered on behalf of firms and clinics and delivered to the media by PR agencies. It is hardly ever possible to check the facts and figures contained in the press releases. The data are at best based on random samples, which are projected onto the whole population. Often enough the claimed number of illness cases relies on random estimates.

No mistrust was voiced when the psychologist Alexander Dröschel from Saarlouis announced to the Germany press agency, dpa, in April of 2002 that approximately 'one million children' between Stralsund and Konstanz were suffering from a psychiatric illness, attention deficit hyperactivity disorder (ADHD). His statement was publicised throughout Germany in spite of the fact that Dröschel had no concrete evidence, as was revealed by my enquiry: 'Greatly varying numbers are circulating. So I picked one out of the middle.'[13] Dröschel's public speculation pleases some pharmaceutical companies: they keep psycho pills ready for fidgeting children so the kids can function in family and school in a better way than nature created them (see Chapter 6). The companies are aggressively courting the young patients' favour. The firm Novartis from Nürnberg has even published a picture book on the subject of ADHD. It makes 'a small white tablet' palatable to the young reader.

One of the companies which invented its own market is Biolitec. 'New trends in cosmetic surgery – successful use of Biolitec lasers for vagina rejuvenation', reported the firm from Jena in August 2002.

'Some clinics in Germany and Austria are already noticeably able to improve the shape of the vagina and to restore a youthful look so as to dramatically increase, among other things, the pleasure-feeling for treated women.'

Of course, there was a lack of proof for the claimed increase in designer-vaginas. When asked about doctors who would laser-embellish vaginas, the representative PR firm, the joint stock company Financial Relations of Frankfurt upon Main, did provide the telephone numbers of two beauty clinics in Reichenhall and Heidelberg. But it turned out that neither establishment had beautified any vaginas. In spite of this, the PR firm wouldn't refute its statement and some days later got hold of a surgeon working in Vienna. The man had 'experience in cosmetic labia correction and confirms the trend'.

Inventing diseases

The invention of diseases knows five forms, detailed by Australian pharmacologists as follows:[14]

Normal life processes are sold as medical problems

Example: Hair loss. When the American firm Merck discovered the first effective remedy for hair growth, the global PR agency Edelman started a campaign. It fed studies to journalists, and a little later one could read, hear and watch: one-third of all men are battling with hair loss. Moreover, an 'International Hair Research Institute' discovered that hair loss was leading to 'panic' as well as 'emotional problems' and diminished the prospect of being successful in job interviews. What was not said: the study is sponsored by Merck and Edelman had found medical experts to dictate quotes to journalists.

Personal and social problems are sold as medical problems

Example: Mental illness. In psychiatry the transformation of the well into the unwell is particularly successful, especially since 'there is no lack of theories', as psychiatrist Klaus Dörner from Hamburg smugly suggests, 'according to which almost all people are mentally ill'.[15] A vivid example has already been mentioned: what was until recently considered to be shyness is called social phobia by the firm Roche, who wants to cure it with an antidepressant. The entrusted advertising agency declared millions of people patients. In addition, conferences and self-help groups have since been sponsored. A journal specialising in marketing describes the campaign as a 'positive example' of how 'public opinion about an illness is being shaped'.

How easy it is to depict the normal state of any human being as a psychiatric illness will be shown in Chapter 5. Asmus Finzen, psychiatrist at the university hospital Basle, says: 'Some psychiatrists indeed go so far with their diagnoses that we are all deemed disturbed in the end.' The number of officially recognised disorders reveals this trend: in the USA, the number of mental illnesses has risen since the Second World War from 26 to 395.

Risks are sold as diseases

Example: Osteoporosis. Pharmaceutical firms sponsored meetings where bone atrophy in older age was declared an illness. Further examples illustrate (in Chapters 3 and 4) how people are persuaded into taking all kinds of examinations. By lowering the norm values of measurable units such as blood pressure or cholesterol level, the circle of sickness is growing. In coming years juggling with risk factors will undergo an unknown acceleration, as a result of the newly decoded human genome. Chapter 10 describes why it is possible to diagnose 'defective' genes in every human being, and how the person concerned – who is in the best of health – is thereby branded as 'not yet sick'.

Rare symptoms are sold as rampant epidemics

Example: Erectile dysfunction. Since the introduction of the potency pill Viagra, impotence is running rampant through the male domain. An Internet site of the Viagra manufacturer Pfizer says: 'Erectile dysfunctions are a serious and common health disorder: Approximately 50 per cent of men between 40 and 70 years are affected – that's every other man.'[16] Hamburg urologist Hartmut Porst, one of the leading potency researchers, thinks that this sweeping statement is exaggerated: 'This is nonsense.'

In a similar way, the pharmaceutical industry is now trying to present frigidity of women as an identifiable and extremely common disease (see page 107): The 'female sexual dysfunction' affects, according to this claim, 43 per cent of all women. Doubtless there are female frigidity problems, but 'the extent is unbelievably exaggerated', says Klaus Diedrich, professor of gynaecology in Lübeck. 'To assume that every other woman has a sexual disorder is a miserable trick.'[17]

Slight symptoms are sold as harbingers of grave disorders

Example: Irritable bowel syndrome (IBS). The phenomenon is accompanied by a profusion of symptoms, which each one of us has experienced at one stage or another and which many of us regard as a normal rumbling in the bowel: aches, diarrhoea and flatulence. '60 to 70 per cent of the population have one or several symptoms of the catalogue of diagnosis criteria, so one is inclined to regard it as abnormal if someone were to be completely free from bother in this regard', argues physician Hermann Füeßl.[18] The vague aches and pains trouble particularly women and have been classed until now as psychosomatic. Only in the course of new drug development was the industry's interest in the alleged illness aroused. What happens during such a phase – behind the high security pharmaceutical fence – only rarely reaches the outside world. Even more revealing therefore is a confidential paper, published in April 2002 by the *British Medical Journal*.[19] It concerns a secret strategy plan drafted by the PR firm In Vivo Communications.[20]

A three-year 'medical education programme' aims, according to the paper, to free the irritable bowel from the bad reputation of a psychosomatic disorder and describe it as a 'credible, common and concrete disease'. The draft concerns the marketing of the drug Alosetron (in the United States: Lotronex) produced by GlaxoSmithKline.

The explicit objective of the training programme it stated: 'IBS, irritable bowel syndrome, must be established in the minds of doctors as a significant and discrete disease state.' Patients also 'need to be convinced that IBS is a common and recognised medical disorder'. The programme's other message is the availability of the new 'clinically proven therapy' Lotronex. The intended first step in its Australian launch was to found a consultancy committee with one important doctor from each Australian state functioning as opinion-maker. In addition, a newsletter was planned to 'establish the market' and to make it clear to gastroenterologists: 'The disease is serious and credible.'

To persuade sceptical general practitioners, In Vivo Communications recommends the publication of articles in leading medical journals, stressing the importance of interviews with opinion-makers. Their contribution is 'invaluable' to make the information appear 'clinically valid'. Pharmacists, nurses, patients and medical associations should be inundated with advertising material. Finally, a 'patient support programme' is to guarantee that GlaxoSmithKline will 'reap the loyalty dividend, when the competitor drug kicks in'. For the success of the project, PR and media activities were, according to In Vivo Communications, 'crucial to a well-rounded campaign particularly in the area of consumer awareness'.

Many of the medical experts and patient groups might have been led by noble motives. The action plan reveals just how insidious the marketing of diseases actually is: apparently independent doctors and organisations who are in fact financed by pharmaceutical firms influence public opinion about a physical or psychological state precisely at the time a new drug is launched onto the market.

The irritable bowel campaign had to be stopped by the way. After the American Food and Drug Administration (FDA) found out about serious side effects, Lotronex was withdrawn from the US market in November 2000. Since June 2002, it has been obtainable again under restricted marketing circulation and stricter control. The FDA pointed out to the manufacturer that 'less than 5 per cent of IBS is considered severe'.[21] In Germany, the active agent has not been licensed.

The example of irritable bowel syndrome is not an exception, but the rule. The British magazine *Pharmaceutical Marketing* advises its readers in a 'practical guide to medical education' how to manage a disease: before the market launch 'a desire' has to be 'created' among medical prescribers and a 'need has to be established'.[22]

Medicalisation as mega trend

Once an invented disease has reached the public conscience, patients and health insurance institutions pay as a matter of course for the appropriate medicaments and therapies. Until now, every reform of the health system failed to put an end to disease mongering – nothing stands in the way of a legally secured exploitation of the social security system, and exploitation also of gullible private patients.

Since the solidarity principle prevails in Germany, no man, woman or child can escape his or her responsibility of funding the health service's expenditure. Every citizen – from baby to pensioner – is paying a daily amount of at least seven Euros into the health system. German health expenditure came to 163.2 billion Euros in 1992 and reached a new record height of 234.2 billion Euros in 2002 – the equivalent of 11.1 per cent of the economy (gross national product).

The price of medicine particularly is on the rise: in Germany costs rose to 32.4 billion in 2000 and have thereby outdone, for the first time, expenditure on medical services. In countries belonging to the Organisation for Economic Cooperation and Development (OECD) – members are the thirty richest nations of the world – the share of public expenditure on pharmaceuticals compared to economic performance rose from 0.4 per cent (1970) to 0.7 per cent in 1996. Behind the deceptively small numbers, a significant increase is hidden: this represents 1.5 per cent points more than average economic growth.

As a result, pharmaceutical firms became bigger and richer. If one applies market capitalisation – the value of an enterprise at the stock exchange – as an indicator, the largest pharmaceutical companies are now competing directly with whole nations. The firm Pfizer comes seventeenth. In other words, it ranks ahead of the 13 million strong Sweden (rank 19) and, for instance, Singapore (rank 39).[23]

The British Nuffield Council on Bioethics, an elite circle of thirteen philosophers, clinicians and scientists, regards the medicalisation of our lives as a mega trend. The worldwide respected think-tank prophesises in a 2002 published report: 'One such problem is that of diagnostic spread, or the tendency for disorders to be broadly defined so that more and more individuals are caught in the diagnostic net.' The council regards profit seeking as the driving force. 'It may be that if medicines are developed that have an effect on a trait, that trait will come to be seen as a disorder, or something to be treated and altered.'[24]

House call to the healthy

It is not only market laws which encourage the expansion of medicine. It also progresses so quickly because the art of healing hasn't seen any major breakthroughs for decades. But where therapies against scourges like cancer fail to materialise, where victories over the spread of AIDS remain elusive, where lucrative pharmaceutical patents expire, where furious research efforts (each day, approximately 5,500 medical articles are published) bring no breakthroughs,[25] medical professionals and pharmaceutical researchers devote their efforts to the hale and hearty.

'Family doctors should also make house calls on the healthy', said a headline of the German *Physicians' Newspaper*.[26] The headline relates to the Heidelberg gerontologist Andreas Kruse. The doctor's intrusion into the private domain is said to help identify health risks. Kruse is getting support from high places for his ruse. Christoph Fuchs, general manager of the Federal Medical Council, backs him up: 'The doctor should not hesitate to check how many bottles of "Klosterfrau Melissengeist" there are in the corner, as this could indicate loneliness, alcohol problems and possibly depression.'

The English medical historian Roy Porter considered the medical-ization of life a structural problem of western health systems and societies due to the fact that the best possible medical care is regarded as a basic right. It manifests as an immense pressure – generated 'by the medical profession, by medi-business, the media, by the high-pressure advertising of pharmaceutical companies, and dutiful (or susceptible) individuals – to expand the diagnosis of treatable illnesses', he says. The fears and interventions were blown up out of proportion, a rocket spiralling out of control. Physicians and consumers were increasingly succumbing to the idea 'that *everyone has something wrong with them, everyone and everything can be cured*'.[27]

What is fair game to some is daylight robbery to others: robbery of their most precious possession – health. The American critic Lynn Payer stated that the activity of the disease mongers gnaws 'away at our self-confidence. And that may make us really sick'. Are we becoming a nation of healthy invalids, incapacitated not by disease, but crippled by imaginary illnesses? The American doctor and author Lewis Thomas was one of the first to warn us of this: 'The new danger to our well-being, if we continue to listen to all the talk, is in becoming a nation of healthy hypochondriacs, living gingerly, worrying ourselves half to death.'[28]

Dr Knock would have been delighted to have such patients. His tragicomic medicine has leapt from the stage into reality. As the *Schweizerische Ärztezeitung* reminded those readers who don't yet know Knock, 'it is almost time to learn from his success story'. The village doctor sets

> a precedent, by developing a promising surgery strategy at a time when neither social security nor marketing seminars were known. Knock takes over a country surgery from his predecessor who had scarcely any patients. In only three months, he develops a mega business, which satisfies everybody involved. In other, or more modern terms: he achieved the classical win-win situation of the free entrepreneur.[29]

2 Myths of medicine

I respect faith, but it is doubt that gets you an education.

Wilson Mizner

Nothing could be more of a turn-off in a publicity campaign than an impotent old man. Yet, Edson Arantes Do Nascimento, better known as Pelé, now over 60, almost passes for sexy. The Brazilian former soccer player is still on form, looks good in a suit and don't forget his love affairs – a decisive credibility enhancer. On posters and in TV adverts since 2002, Pelé raises a problem nobody likes to talk about: 'Erection disorder. Talk to your doctor – I would.'

The campaign, for which Pelé is said to have received a six-figure amount from American pharmaceutical firm Pfizer, is interesting in two regards. First, the fit football pensioner does not have, as he assures us, any problems with limpness. His problem lies with abstinence: Pelé has, at last count, fathered four children by two wives and has at least another two daughters from extramarital affairs.

Second, it is amazing that Pelé makes no mention at all of the potency pill Viagra that his sponsor produces. That is exactly why Pelé's campaign on male potency is such a brilliant example of the pharmaceutical industry's latest marketing trick: it is not for drugs that the drums are played, but rather the *diseases* being advertised. In magazines and on advertising pillars eye-catching messages warn us that we might have diminished potency, depression or fungus.

Pelé, a messenger of Viagra manufacturer Pfizer, cares – seemingly out of love for his neighbour – generally and genuinely for the vanishing virility of his male mates. The limpness of the penis, erectile dysfunction, is extremely widespread, announces the international star. 'Fear and inhibition prevent many men from talking to their doctor about erectile problems', Pfizer prompts Pelé to say.[1]

Pharmaceutical company Wyeth, just another example, promotes the clinical picture of depression. Under the heading '"Pleasure" Check List' it placed an advert in the magazine *Nurse* to track down potential patients.[2] The text reads:

Life does not always give you what you're hoping for. You might feel disappointed – and often on a low. If the low persists, all joy vanishes. And, in the long run, a joyless life can make you ill. Take your personal test. Right now.

Then a questionnaire follows:

1 Have you lost interest in your relationship or can't you enjoy it as you used to?
2 Do you find it difficult to take your mind off worries and fears that are related to partnership and loneliness?
3 Has your weight or appetite significantly increased or decreased lately?
4 Do you have difficulty falling asleep or sleeping through the night?
5 Has your interest in sex decreased lately or have you lost your sexual appetite?
6 Do you have the feeling that friends are starting to turn away from you?
7 Do you often feel worthless?

Anybody who answers yes to four out of the seven questions seems to be ready for therapy, according to the pharmaceutical firm, and should 'talk to a male or female doctor in confidence'.

Serious psychiatrists reject the questionnaire. Peter Riedesser, head of the department for child and adolescent psychiatry and psychotherapy at the university clinic Hamburg-Eppendorf, says: 'The checklist shows where the pharma firms' journey is heading: directly to the end consumers, so that they, in turn, can then influence the medical body.'

Pharmaceutical firms would like to advertise their pills directly to the consumer. This, however, is not allowed for prescription medicine within the European Union. Consequentially, the afore-mentioned 'Disease Awareness Campaigns' were born. These often global advertising crusades are aimed at making people aware that certain diseases do exist – with the idea of selling the appropriate medicines and therapies to them as a second stage.

This indirect form of advertising medicines is gaining popularity in the pharmaceutical industry. On poster walls, in magazine adverts and on the Internet, drug producers plant the seeds in people's minds that they might be ill and in need of treatment. The year '2001 has witnessed a rising number of pharma companies turning to public education initiatives [to build on the growing global trend of patient empowerment]', says marketing expert Chris Ross. 'The informed patient is fast becoming a focal point of big pharma's marketing strategies.'[3]

These Disease Awareness Campaigns are only a small part of the litany that wants to talk us out of our health. The role of the prayer leaders falls to the disease mongers: they preach to us about ever-new symptoms and syndromes, which allegedly endanger our mental and physical well-being.

Much of what we are served as a new threat or a sensational therapy is based on the alleged progress of modern medicine. However, mistrust and scepticism are appropriate: from clinical research to medical laity, the supposed news has to travel a long way, and people who by profession take great interest in falsifying and twisting messages on health issues line this road. Researchers, journalists, physicians and employees of pharmaceutical firms cannot always withstand the temptation.

The advice of the house doctor, the article in the prestigious specialist magazine, the brochure of the pharmaceutical firm and the medical article in the daily newspaper – before information reaches us, much has been concealed, modified or added. How this manipulation of medicine happens will be described in the following section.

Pharmaceutical industry aims at physicians

Physicians, who normally want to help others, now experience themselves in the care of others. For every single doctor the pharmaceutical industry is spending 8,000 to 13,000 Euros a year on marketing measures, so that he or she prescribes the pills and products of the respective firm. Medical practitioners and hospital consultants are completely overrun by representatives of the industry. The GlaxoSmithKline enterprise alone employs in Europe and the USA an army of 17,000 pharmaceutical advisers. The total number of all pill sales representatives increased in the United States between 1996 and 2001 by 110 per cent: it rose from 42,000 to 88,000 pharmaceutical advisers.

Because of such enormous demand, the limited time that a doctor can spend with the many and largely uninvited visitors can actually be sold. This business is done for example by the firm Time Concepts with its headquarters in the US state of Kentucky. For a fee of 105 dollars, it arranges a ten-minute meeting between pharmaceutical adviser and doctor. Time Concepts pockets 50 dollars of the amount, another 50 dollars go to the doctor who, on top of this, can choose a favourite charity – to it the remaining 5 dollars are donated.[4]

The payment system of Time Concepts seems more honest than the usual practice: with dinner invitations, travel expenses to exotic conference venues and other privileges, the pill and equipment sellers are courting the doctors' favour. Even medical students in their final terms receive presents from pharmaceutical companies. Junior doctors in American teaching hospitals are almost daily invited for lunch, even though pizza is often on the menu. Doctors who attend industry seminars can expect to be treated to a meal in a high-class restaurant.

The transition from legal marketing to illegal favouritism is well underway. At 'gas-and-go', doctor and adviser meet at the petrol station. The pharmaceutical representative is able to present his or her products and then pays the doctor's petrol bill.[5] In 2002, the public prosecutors' office in Munich opened preliminary inquiries into thousands of German hospital doctors and employees of the SmithKlineBeecham concern.

The public prosecutors who confiscated numerous documents at the firm's headquarters in Munich's Leopold Street stirred suspicion of the granting and accepting of advantage as well as bribery and aiding and abetting tax evasion. According to documents from travel agencies, doctors had accepted invitations to the finals of the 1998 football championship in Paris and to Formula One races. In addition, the pharmaceutical firm had allegedly paid for books and computers.

Such scandals surface from time to time to fill the general public with outrage and nourish the cliché of the 'fleecers in white'. However, doctors who admit to 'selling themselves' directly to the industry are the exception. Much more widespread and therefore more alarming are those insidious practices that the industry uses to influence doctors in their everyday work. The proximity of pharmaceutical firms and medical practitioners is nowadays accepted as a matter of course.

An example: most of the statutory further education for physicians in Germany is openly organised by the pharmaceutical industry. Only a fraction of the events are officially regarded as independent. It appears, however, that even in these few cases, drug producers are in fact also involved, as was shown by an inquiry led by Dr Peter Sawicki, head of department at a Cologne hospital, and two colleagues of the North Rhine Academy for Further Medical Education. In thirty-two out of the fifty-one examined events it turned out. that firms like Roche, Bayer, Pfizer and Hoechst were indeed involved in the supposedly independent seminars.

Pens and writing pads with advertising imprints were ready for the doctors, during the breaks they were offered snacks and drinks by the firms and later on, a hot evening meal was served in half of all the events. Peter Sawicki doubts that the appearance of pharmaceutical people will have no consequences: 'It is feared in this context that the selection of consultants and event topics is being influenced by market economic interests of the involved industry.'[6]

With kind regards from the industry

The progress of medicine has reached gigantic dimensions so that only a very few physicians are able to penetrate the jungle of possible diagnoses and therapies. Because of this, medical guidelines were introduced, supposedly to facilitate better knowledge. These guidelines are – often after tough negotiations – formulated by medical experts and intended to allow the large mass of less specialised colleagues to practise according to the latest scientific knowledge.

When guidelines happen to recommend a certain drug therapy, the drug manufacturer is practically receiving a blank cheque, and the state even encourages the producer to cash it. All the more serious then is what a group around Dr Allan Detsky from Mount Sinai Hospital in Toronto found out: medical guidelines are, to an alarming degree, subject to the industry's influence. For their study, the researchers contacted 192 guideline authors in Europe and North America and asked them whether they had connections to the pharmaceutical industry. Significantly, nearly half of the doctors preferred to refrain from answering.

Exactly one hundred of the answers received could be analysed and evaluated: 87 per cent of the guideline writers had general connections to the pharmaceutical industry; 59 per cent were linked to the firms whose products they were recommending in the guidelines; 38 per cent were consultants or direct employees of pharmaceutical companies; 6 per cent were shareholders of firms. And among all evaluated guidelines not a single one was found that was written independently of drug manufacturers. 'In conclusion, there appears to be a high degree of interaction between authors of clinical practice guidelines and the pharmaceutical industry', Allan Detsky states laconically. He fears: 'These specific interactions may influence the practice of a very large number of physicians.'

The critics are demanding something that should actually be a matter of course, or so it seems: in future, all authors' conflicts of interests should be noted in the medical guidelines. And doctors with significant conflicts of interests should generally be excluded from writing guidelines. Only, which degree of connection is significant and which isn't? Detsky knows how difficult it is to draw the line. He asks ironically, 'Is there a threshold, below which authors will not perceive subconscious influences from their relationships with pharmaceutical companies?'[7]

The illusion of incorruptible research

Interconnections between commerce and the art of healing run through the whole medical complex: doctors give advice to medicine producers and test their active agents in clinical studies. They are members of 'Advisory Boards', those apparently independent committees that take action at the right moment, precisely when medicines are launched onto the market. Doctors could become dependent, fears Martina Dören, professor for women's health at the Free University Berlin. She says:

> Because the funding of scientific expert societies, based on members' contributions, is as a general rule rather sparse, it has unfortunately become an established fact that conferences cannot be held anymore without substantial financial support from pharmaceutical firms.[8]

Basle psychiatrist Asmus Finzen follows the liaison between healers and dealers with growing unease. Medical researchers

> appear as permanent consultants at firm symposiums, trade as authors of publications that are written by the firms' ghost-writers and support certain medicines or equipments at firm-sponsored events. They accept expensive gifts and have their luxury travel financed. They conclude patents and share contracts and are holders of company shares or options

complained Finzen in the journal *Deutsches Ärzteblatt*. He went on to write, 'Certainly, not all medical researchers liaise with the industry in this kind of way. But there are many.'[9]

In industrialised countries, it is quite usual that medical professors and medical practitioners speak at press conferences on behalf of enterprises and pocket high fees. Employees of pharmaceutical firms are frequently searching for medical doctors who are prepared to appear in public to promote the firm for a fee – such recruitment is called 'opinion leader management' or 'opinion-maker monitoring'. Before the start of an event, the doctors have to show the pharmaceutical representatives which slides they are intending to show during their lectures. During these 'slide reviews' it might happen that 'the firm wants to take half of the slides out of the lecture', reports Hamburg urologist Hartmut Porst.

I sing the song of the one whose bread I eat

When one confronts doctors with the suggestion that their financial connections to the industry might influence their work and judgement, they completely reject the idea. As scientists they were able to preserve their objectivity, doctors say, for this reason it was irrelevant who finances their research. 'Physicians . . . deny industry's influence, even when such enticements as all-expenses-paid trips to luxury resorts are provided', says bio-ethicist Susan Coyl. In an extensive study, she described the pharmaceutical industry's influence on medical doctors on behalf of the American Society for Internal Medicine. According to her analysis, the independence of the doctors is suffering: 'Research shows a strong correlation between receiving industry benefits and favouring their products.'[10]

A group under the supervision of Henry Stelfox from the University of Toronto proved the same phenomenon for the case of a controversial drug (calcium-channel antagonists). The researchers read seventy publications on the subject and divided them into three categories: critical, neutral or supportive. Then they approached the publications' authors per questionnaire to find out whether and to what extent they had received money from the industry. The result was only too clear: every author who had written positively about the medicine had received money from the industry in one way or another. In 96 per cent of the cases, the drug supporters had received financial subsidies from the producer of the respective drug. By comparison only 37 per cent of the critical doctors had accepted money from the industry.[11]

The disease dealers' strongest currency is in medical journals' published studies that seem to prove the benefit of the specific drug. These reports are often the crucial factor in deciding whether a new substance will be licensed. Moreover, they contribute to the decision about whether and to what extent the doctors will later on rely on the new medicament.

These seemingly objective technical articles are in many cases subject to the pharmaceutical industry's influence. Medical doctor Lisa Kjaergard from the University Hospital in Copenhagen has examined 159 technical articles from twelve branches of medicine with the following findings: when researchers work on behalf of the industry, they judge the researched treatment method beneficially more often than average.[12]

One study, published by Californian doctor Thomas Bodenheimer in the *New England Journal of Medicine*, reveals also the clear, sometimes blatant influence of the industrial sponsors on clinical studies: pharmaceutical firms repress, embellish and alter the results of studies, which they commission originally independent researchers to carry out. Six out of twelve researchers whom Bodenheimer interviewed admitted that their work had been subject to influence. Either the unfavourable results of studies – from the viewpoint of the commissioner – were not published at all or they were manipulated.

In one case, the pharmaceutical firm delayed the publication of results, demanding amendments. 'During the delay, the company secretly wrote a competing article on the same topic, which was favourable to the company's viewpoint', says Bodenheimer. Another researcher discovered side effects of a drug and described them in a draft he gave the firm. As a result, the critical doctor received threats that his work would never receive grants again. Moreover, the firm published its own report that gave the side effects only fleeting mention.

In another case, the tested substance was, according to the researching doctors, completely ineffective. The commissioning party, apparently, did not have a different view – and the article disappeared quietly into the back of a drawer. Such unbecoming manoeuvres, however, are only rarely required. For most of the time, according to Bodenheimer's investigations, medical studies would be planned in advance in such a way as to present the respective products in the most favourable light. One of the affected doctors complained: 'Industry control over [test] data allows companies to provide the spin on the data that favours them.'[13]

At the annual conference of the European Society for Cardiology 2001 in Stockholm, Dutch heart expert Marteen Simons complained publicly about his financers from the medicine industry. One company had urged him 'not to publicise unnecessarily any data that could lead to economic disadvantages for the enterprise'.[14]

In view of such a state of affairs, a withdrawal of the pharmaceutical industry from clinical research would be desirable. But it is not expected. On the contrary, the coffers of public hospitals, university clinics and state research institutes are empty. Medical doctors are nowadays more than ever before dependent on funds from industry and sponsorship to keep research up and running.

Even the elite of German science has formed an alliance with a pharmaceutical multinational. The Max Planck Society, funded by tax money, founded a research laboratory in October 2002 in Munich together with the GlaxoSmithKline enterprise. The 'Genetic Research Centre' is situated in the grounds of the Max Planck Institute for Psychiatry in Munich, and subsidised by GlaxoSmithKline with a contribution that amounts to millions of Euros.

In return for this, the pharmaceutical researchers gain access to a treasure which otherwise they would not have been able to buy for any money in the world: a unique collection of human tissue samples. Max Planck researchers under psychiatrist Florian Holsboer are actually on the track of the biological foundations of depression. They have examined proteins in the brain fluid, analysed stress hormones in the blood, measured electrical currents in hundreds of depressed people's brains and thereby gathered a data collection which is unique in the world.

At the laboratory – half pharmaceutical firm and half Max Planck Institute – it will be important to separate strictly economic and scientific interests. Otherwise, the industry could influence which direction the research at the state-owned Max Planck Institute will be heading.

Pharmaceutical companies regularly entrust academic researchers with the task of examining the benefit and safety of medicaments. MDs at university clinics demand high fees and are comparably critical – that is why pharmaceutical firms are currently changing direction; they prefer to give private companies the job of carrying out clinical studies. Only 40 per cent of the industry's research funds goes to academic scientists, 60 per cent goes nowadays to private companies – the latter figure has tripled within a decade.

A less than transparent multimillion business has emerged. Pharmaceutical concerns entrust hundreds of specialised test firms, which in turn cooperate with many thousands of practising doctors. The latter recruit test persons from the waiting room and pocket head premiums for the service. The swift access to a single test subject is, for drug manufacturers in the United States, worth between 2,000 and 5,000 dollars.[15] In Germany the tariff ranges from 1,500 to 1,700 Euros per study participant, says Hartmut Porst, who carries out clinical studies with potency pills on patients of his surgery for urology in Hamburg.

The boom of private commissioned research will increase concerns about the influence on clinical studies even further, warns a group of ethicists from the American Medical Association. The entrusted private companies 'might encounter considerable conflicts of interest because they are paid by pharmaceutical companies that ultimately depend on positive trial outcomes'.[16]

Some drug studies are not carried out to clarify scientific questions, but they are solely performed to place a medicament onto the market. Dutch investigator Hans ter Steege from the public health department in The Hague looked into so-called application studies. These should serve to clarify any outstanding scientific questions after the licensing of a medicament. However, in two-thirds of the studies, as Hans ter Steege's inquiries showed, the firms were explicitly pursuing a different objective: namely, establishing their pills on the market.

The ploy works as follows: the medical practitioner recruits among his or her regular patients test persons and prescribes them the respective medication. For this service the enterprise pays the medical practitioner a certain amount of money. In return, the pharmaceutical companies get doctors and patients accustomed to the new medication – so accustomed that they continue to prescribe and take it, long after the alleged study has run out.[17]

The myth of the informed patient

In their profit seeking, pharmaceutical companies do not only influence doctors and clinical researchers. They are increasingly turning directly towards potential customers in efforts to arouse in them the need for medical treatment. The German Federal Association of the Pharmaceutical Industry has offered seminars to self-help groups to educate them in the ways of public relations. In an insidious way, the industry is roping in groups of affected individuals to make diseases known throughout the entire population.

A report of the Boston Consulting Group recommends that pharmaceutical enterprises systematically seek the proximity of the consumer: 'Companies can drive demand, by providing continuous, targeted support for each consumer decision point.' The report promises the medical industry rosy prospects: in the future, therapies would 'become available for previously untreated health and quality-of-life conditions'.[18]

The Internet is providing pharmaceutical firms with an ideal medium to 'integrate the patient more actively', as consultancy firm A. T. Kearney in Düsseldorf puts it.[19] Disease Awareness Campaigns are supported by hosts of Internet sites that inform the consumer about the alleged illnesses. Patient organisations and medical associations also communicate on the Internet – their sites too are often sponsored by pharmaceutical companies.

For an American concern, A. T. Kearney developed a 'direct patient access strategy'. Through brochures, Internet portals and call centres, the concern is supposed to obtain direct patient access. Interestingly, this access should not only be limited to the realm of physical medicine, but also reach psychological and lifestyle issues.

This way the pharmaceutical concern would gain some kind of permanent line directly to the customer. If German laws one day would allow it, A. T. Kearney says, prescription drugs could be dispensed directly through the connections put in place. While the pharmaceutical industry would then take care of the patient via the Internet, the treating doctor could concentrate in the surgery on his or her 'actual task' – the only remaining question would then be of what this task would actually consist.

The beautiful and the sick

Well-known people are particularly useful for bringing diseases to the public's attention. Not always do they make such a public appearance as potent Pelé or the Bavarian prime minister's wife, Karin Stoiber, who acted in October 2002 as patron of the World Osteoporosis Day in Munich. American PR agent Amy Domer Schachtel has made a profession out of harnessing celebrities very discreetly to the pharmaceutical industry's cart. The well-known faces talk in public about lesser known diseases – many of these celebrities pocket fees for this. 'The trend is growing dramatically', says Schachtel, who runs her firm Premier Entertainment from a residence in New Jersey.[20]

Schachtel's protégés have succeeded in reaching top TV programmes in the United States. In the *Today Show*, the famous US sitcom star Kelsey Grammer and his wife were chatting about irritable bowel syndrome. The actor Cybill Shepherd revealed to talk show host Oprah Winfrey and her millions-strong audience which antidote she is taking for menopausal troubles.

Hollywood stars like Kathleen Turner and Lauren Bacall have also been chatting on American TV about their aches and pains – neither the viewers nor the station suspected they were being paid for this by the pharmaceutical industry. Kathleen Turner, who talked about her struggle against arthritis, received money from firms Amgen and Wyeth. The news channel CNN has recently started taking notion against this type of 'surreptitious' advertising: prominent figures are asked about their financial connections before they are allowed to chat about their health in front of the camera.[21]

Advertising – until the patient turns up

The pharmaceutical lobby is urging the European Union to give it permission to advertise its drugs directly to the consumer. As far as prescription drugs are concerned, this is still prohibited – for a good reason, as a glance at the USA reveals. In 1997, the licensing agency FDA made it considerably easier to advertise drugs. Exact information about the side effects of medicaments can now be omitted. Since the deterrent small print has disappeared from pharmaceutical advertisements, the number of campaigns for prescription drugs has rocketed.

Only rarely do the pharmaceutical adverts deal with serious illnesses. As a rule they stalk those in the grey zone between sick and healthy. In this state, as medical doctor Lisa Schwartz from Dartmouth Medical School in Hanover (New Hampshire) found, people could be persuaded they had certain conditions. Together with colleagues, she scientifically analysed sixty-seven different drug adverts in ten popular American magazines like *Time*, *People* or *Good Housekeeping*. The result of her analysis sounds strangely familiar:

> Our findings suggest that most prescription drugs advertised to consumers target common symptoms (e.g., sneezing, hair loss, being overweight), which many patients would have managed without a physician. Although a pharmacological approach might be appropriate for some, the danger is that by turning ordinary experiences into diagnoses – by designating a runny nose as allergic rhinitis – the boundaries of medicine might become unreasonably broad.

Hence the advertising messages were promoting medicalisation in an almost perfect way, warns Lisa Schwartz. The very moment a consumer lets the doctor prescribe him or her a medicament, his or her condition becomes a symptom: 'The affected person is now a patient.'[22]

US citizens watch a daily average of nine TV advertisements for medicines.[23] In 1999, the industry spent US$1.8 billion on publicity.

In Germany, the antidepressant Paxil alone was advertised in 2000 with a budget of 91.8 million Marks. Consequently, sales on the hotly contested US pharmaceutical market rose by 25 per cent and catapulted the alleged happiness pill into eighth place among the best-selling drugs.[24]

With rising advertisement budgets in the United States, the number of people whose undermined self-confidence makes them run to the doctor is on the rise as well. Some 20 per cent of all adult US citizens contact a doctor because of pharmaceutical advertisements, as a representative survey among 25,182 people showed.[25]

Journalists lend a hand

The media have become an important tool of the pharmaceutical industry. In editorial departments, invitations to industry-sponsored seminars, symposia and workshops arrive day in and day out. Add to this tons of press releases and brochures. As a rule, sponsors pay travel and hotel expenses, just to make sure that journalists arrive at the venue.

Boat trips on Hamburg's Alster in the summer are as much a part of press events as wine tasting, cigar soirées and formal dinners. In February 2003, the firm Dr Kade/Besins held a press conference in Hamburg to present its new testosterone gel. The supporting programme delighted journalists: it was, according to the invitation, an 'exclusive cookery course accompanied by food tasting and wine sampling' at the exquisite Le Canard restaurant.

The company Lilly-Icos splashed out as well when it presented its new potency pill at the Hamburg Congress Centrum in December 2002. Afterwards, journalists were invited to a 'fairy-tale dinner à la 1001 Nights – Syrian specialities in oriental ambiance'.

Access to journalists is a highly sought after merchandise, for which physicians and pharmaceutical companies pay PR firms a high price. 'We make sure you're in the press' – thus advertises Hamburg agency Impressum, which works for a number of medical associations. To do that, it brings its connections with editorial staff to bear and carries out press work for conferences. In one of Impressum's brochures, it says:

> Through our publicity work and personal contacts we attained, depending on the size of a conference, a participation rate of 50 to 350 journalists. Consequently, we achieved coverage per

conference of up to 500 reports in the press as well as on radio and TV.

Many of the launched stories are adopted and circulated by journalists without question. Possible therapies are rashly broadcasted to the public as supposed sensations – later, in most of the cases, their fleeting notoriety dwindles into obscurity. The tendency to exaggerate is an occupational hazard that affects many medical journalists. They often sensationalise the spread of certain diseases and their potential threat, to make their reporting appear relevant and important.

The extent of misinformation in medical journalism has received sparse systematic examination until now. It is therefore rewarding to look at a study published in June 2000 by Harvard Medical School.[26] The four authors examined articles and reports on three medicaments that had been published in leading American media: the *Wall Street Journal*, the *New York Times*, the *Washington Post* and thirty-three other American newspapers as well as the four TV stations ABC, CBS, CNN and NBC.

All in all, the scientists examined 207 contributions. The result of the Harvard analysis is sobering: in 40 per cent of all contributions, data and figures about the claimed effect of the medicament were missing, so that readers or viewers were unable to assess the drug's benefit for themselves. Among the 124 stories that had provided quantitative information, 83 per cent reported only on the relative benefit – a widespread bad practice that can easily mislead the reader or viewer.

One example: a CBS film on osteoporosis reported that a new medication would reduce the risk of hip fractures by 50 per cent. The reporter described this figure as being 'almost miraculous' – while it was in fact relating to the *relative* risk. In *absolute* figures, the miracle seems far more modest: out of a hundred people who had not taken the drug, *two* suffered a bone fracture. In the comparative group, *one* person suffered a fracture. This means the drug has reduced the appearance of fractures among the test persons from 2 to 1 per cent.

The many side effects of the three drugs (Aspirin, cholesterol reducer Pravastatin and osteoporosis drug Alendronat) received no mention at all in 53 per cent of the stories. And finally, in 61 per cent of the reports any financial connections the quoted experts had to the respective drug producers were concealed.

An 'effective educational programme' for medical journalists is necessary, demand the Harvard researchers, for them to produce reports that are more balanced. But do they even want this? The mockery, that medical journalists thrive on fanning the flames of hypochondria among people by incessantly sounding the alarm because of this or that disease, surely contains some grains of truth. The supposed bad news of disease mongers is good news for the media.

3 A disease called diagnosis

A healthy person has been examined the wrong way.

Medics' slogan

Travelling healers are roaming the country. They are driving futuristic vehicles and do not demand money for their services. On market squares and churchyards, they drag people into their vehicles, give them a thorough check-up – and finally release many of them converted into patients. The chalk-white 'Osteoporosis research mobile' went on tour for the first time in Germany, from northern Hamburg to southern Erfurt, in the summer of 2002. Women over 60 are lured into the conveyance for a thorough medical check-up including bone density measurement. This is the way citizens suffering from age-related bone atrophy, the so-called osteoporosis, are tracked down. The search for sick women was not free from self-interest. It was sponsored by a foundation – and by fourteen pharmaceutical companies and producers of medical products.[1]

Men are also plagued: by employees of the Pfizer firm, who tour in a blue and white lorry through approximately thirty German cities. 'The Healthy Man' is written in big letters on the truck. The payload area is extendable, to triple its ground size. Inside there are five examination cubicles as well as an 'information bar'. In the truck, curious onlookers and passers-by get a medical in ten minutes. Medically trained technical staff measure cholesterol level, blood sugar, blood pressure and weight. 'If the man doesn't go to the check-up, the check-up must come to the man', runs Pfizer's credo. On the margin of a big golf tournament, for example, 6,297 normal men were processed through the diagnosis vehicle. And there you have it: half of the examined had elevated blood pressure and 44 per cent showed abnormal blood test results.

The osteoporosis mobile and the Pfizer truck seem to be harbingers of medical practice that seeks to infiltrate the whole of society. Like travelling docs and quacks in medieval times, disease mongers are nowadays out there to hunt down patients. That they are succeeding in tracking down seemingly ill people everywhere is in the nature of the game. It is true that Germans are perky and living longer than ever before in the history of the country; the healthy Teutons, however, are not living up to the standards of modern healing science. That is because the medical risk factors are deliberately defined so as to ensure that everybody may have something wrong with them.

And that's how it works. A laboratory result is obtained by using a large number of healthy people, for example blood donors, recruits and sport students. As a next step, the average of the measured results is calculated. Those 95 per cent in the middle are arbitrarily defined as 'normal levels'. The 5 per cent of outsiders drawn from either side are classified, however, as 'anomalous' – although the people from whom the values were obtained are completely healthy.[2] Consequently, one could depict the whole of humanity as sick: if a certain laboratory value is abnormal in every 5 per cent of the population, the percentage of the anomalies will rise with every new examination. After twenty measured values, for example, only 36 per cent of people remain healthy all over. And after a hundred, the figure is as low as less than 1 per cent.[3] From this, physicians have drawn the conclusion that a healthy person is one who has not or not yet been examined thoroughly enough.

Some risk factors have been fixed in advance so as to net not only 5 per cent, but also complete cross-sections of the population. For cholesterol, just to mention an example, the limits were defined in Germany a few years ago, so that people with 'normal' values are in the minority, whereas those with 'abnormal' values represent the majority.

But how can that be? A comprehensive study of 100,000 people in Bavaria showed a mean value of 6.7 millimoles per litre (mmol/l) or 260 milligram per decilitre (mg/dl) of blood. The 'National Cholesterol Initiative', a private interest group of thirteen medical professors, however, proposed in 1990 a 5.2 millimole or 200 milligram limit and was successful. The medics of the cholesterol initiative represented lobby groups, including the industry-aligned German League for the Fight against High Blood Pressure as well as the Lipid-League and the German Society for Laboratory Medicine. In a 'strategy paper', they demanded the aggressive expansion of therapy: 'Every medical practitioner should know the cholesterol level of his or her patient.'[4]

By degree of financially interested medical doctors, the majority of Germans have been auth... at risk. In the age group of 30 to 39 year olds, 68 per cent of men and 56 per cent of women have, according to the arbitrary limit, a pathologically elevated cholesterol level. In the age group of 50 to 59 year olds, it is even higher: 84 per cent of men and 93 per cent of women.

In the United States the National Heart, Lung, and Blood Institute issued in July 2004 guidelines that recommend lowering the threshold for treating the 'bad cholesterol' (low density lipoprotein) levels from 3.4 mmol/l (130 mg/dl) to 2.6 mmol/l (100 mg/dl) for individuals without heart disease. While the effect is unproven, these new guidelines, which were endorsed by the American Heart Association, are likely to have radically increased the number of people taking cholesterol-lowering drugs.[5] The guidelines sparked a furore when it was shown that all but one of the nine authors had financial ties to the manufacturers of cholesterol-lowering drugs. It was only subsequently that the National Heart, Lung, and Blood Institute revealed on its websites these financial interests.[6]

The absurd result of such thresholds is that the alleged risk patients feel healthy and fit. If they were suffering from anything at all, then it must be the anomalous diagnosis. Viennese satirist Karl Kraus was right then: diagnosis is the most common disease.

Pointless check-up makes patients happy

Since October 1989, a general medical examination, the so-called 'check-up', has existed in Germany. Every medically insured person over 35 has the right to have a complete examination every two years at the expense of the public health system. To create enthusiasm for the check-up, the Federal Association of Public Health Insurance Scheme Doctors organised, at the beginning of 1991, a nationwide education campaign. The motto was 'Better to live longer happily'.

However, whether the mass screening of the healthy brings any benefit has not been proven. The only certainty is that it provides the medics of public health with a very welcome income source. Uwe Heyll, specialist for internal medicine, Düsseldorf, judges: 'In the case of the check-up one has to fear that the commitment of doctors to this preventive service was primarily lead by commercial considerations.' An article from the business section of the *Physicians' Newspaper* in 1991 is also revealing:

If a surgery had among its clientele just 1,000 patients, who were entitled to claim, it would be possible to realise an additional turn-over of circa 70,000 D-Mark every two years, that is 35,000 Mark per year. Roughly 3,000 Mark per month. A figure, which can be increased, if cancer prevention is done at the same time. Marvellous![7]

Two years after introducing the check-up, public health doctors tried to prove its benefit. They presented statistics which made them deeply happy: only 43 per cent of the examined people had escaped *without* a diagnosis, while 57 per cent were caught in medicine's net. And of course, the percentage of those at risk can be increased – as we have seen – by adding further tests. 'In a few years time, except for those who do not participate in the check-up, hardly anybody will be considered healthy any more', prophesies Uwe Heyll.[8]

It should give us much food for thought that the United States' most important medical societies have been demanding, for quite a while now, that check-ups be abolished. Because they do not give the examined people any benefit, US medics would prefer to spend money on other, more effective measures. The only problem is that the preventive examination cannot now be abolished. Patients have grown fond of the medically superfluous check-up and would rebel against its discontinuation.[9]

Picture fury approved by health insurance scheme

On 16 January 1896, *The New York Times* printed the coarse-grained photo of a woman's hand. It showed bones surrounded by the half shadow of tissue. The public stared unbelievingly at the first X-ray image. Since this first image, taken by physics professor Wilhelm Conrad Roentgen from Würzburg (who, by the way, looked through his wife's hand), pictures have unleashed a revolutionary change in medicine. Nowadays, it is possible to look into the human body at millimetre range. Physicians can detect bone fractures or tumours effortlessly, it seems, and plan complicated operations on screen.

At major clinics the picture archive grows daily by one cubic metre, and around 1.8 million computer tomographs are shot every year in Germany alone. The picture fury in medicine cannot be solely explained by seeking knowledge. The 'iconomania' of medicine, as internist Linus S. Geisler from Gladbeck called the phenomenon, leads also to an alarmingly high number of wrong results and superfluous diagnoses. 'Essential elements of today's X-ray screenings . . .

are superfluous', criticised the Expert Council for Concerted Action in the Health System, an independent body that advises the German Federal Ministry of Health. Up to one hundred X-ray images exist of some of our contemporaries, and the pictures tend to accumulate during the last months of life. For patients with back pain, imaging procedures are also used quite indiscriminately.

Because of the increasingly more precise image diagnostic, medical experts happen upon pathological results, which nevertheless allow one to grow very old. Neurologist Frithjof Kruggel of the Max Planck Institute for Neuropsychological Research in Leipzig, Germany says: 'Some of the things one comes across would formerly only have been discovered on the dissection table.'[10]

Here come the body scanners

A glaring excrescence of X-ray medicine is currently spreading in the United States. All over the country, more than a hundred centres have emerged where healthy people choose to have a complete body scan, just for prevention. Within only ten minutes, computer tomographs (CT) provide three-dimensional total body images of the client's insides. The procedure is painless, but it comes with the inconvenience of potentially harmful exposure to X-rays.

In the search for pathological signs, the doctor can comb methodically through the stack of tomograms: from top to toe, cut into millimetre-thin slices, the body emerges on screen. Some of the 2 million dollar CT devices are set up in shopping malls. In California the body scanners are even rolling through towns and cities in enormous trucks, always looking out for the imaginary sick and the fearful healthy. 'I want to be around to see my son grow up', says building contractor William Shuford, an entirely healthy man who handed over 800 dollars for the privilege of climbing into the BodyScan Company's CT tube in Orlando, Florida.

Whether the total body scan gives him an advantage is a scientifically unproven matter. A result that gives no cause for concern is still no guarantee that a tumour would not erupt after all, that the heart would not fail or an artery not clog up any time soon. What one is most likely to lose in the CT tube is the pleasant sensation of feeling healthy – in almost everybody, the scanners find at least a small thing, even if it is most often harmless. A shadow on the lung, for example, can be the harmless scar of a previous inflammation – which the patient finds out only by enduring expensive follow-up examinations. For these reasons, the Association of American X-ray

Doctors refuses to body-scan trouble-free people. Radiologist James Borgstede explains: 'The scans may cause unnecessary worry and expense, and could give a false sense of security.'[11]

The human brain is also being scanned up to the very last blind spot. By nuclear magnetic resonance imaging doctors hope to discover schizophrenia, Alzheimer's and other diseases of the intellectual organ in their earliest stages. In a decade, thus forecasts Dennis Selkoe of Harvard Medical School, doctors would scan human brain health by imaging procedures as a matter of course, comparable to present-day cholesterol level tests.

Medical jargon camouflages ignorance

For the medical industry, diagnosis is the foundation of business and at the same time the first link in the value chain. A healthy person would undermine the whole system – therefore he or she is in need of a diagnosis. Tirelessly, organisations such as the industry-supported Hochdruckliga (High-Blood-Pressure League) or the Bundesverband der Niedergelassenen Kardiologen (Federal Association of Practising Cardiologists) call upon healthy people to give in to care prevention. The check-up results in laboratories declare millions of healthy people sick.

Without a doubt, diagnosis is indispensable for medicine. The physician needs it to establish order in the welter of diseases. Only if doctors recognise an ailment can they use their experience, consult medical books and exchange opinions with colleagues. Diagnoses inform the patient and tell clinicians who is to be treated and how.

But the trouble is, healthy people too are often tagged with a diagnosis as soon as they enter an examination room. In about half the cases of people consulting the family doctor, no biological disease can be proven. This is a situation with which the health system cannot live: insurance claim forms, national health schemes and pension providers demand that a diagnosis be put onto paper. Doctors cannot examine a person without committing themselves to a certain diagnosis afterwards, because it has to be written down on the health insurance claim.

Hence, diagnoses are often no more than hot air. Doctors construct illnesses by 'solely relying on the symptoms described by the patient', argues Uwe Heyll from the University of Düsseldorf. 'Such a diagnosis is of course no more than speculation, but it is enough to fulfil its function' – namely to satisfy patient and doctor, and probably drug companies as well, if they can come up with a remedy for the invented condition

With Greek and Latin medical terms, doctors camouflage their ignorance. 'Coital cephalgia' for example is nothing more than a headache during intercourse, and the scientifically dressed up word for a slight pain in the anus is 'proctalgia fugax'. 'Similarly a nosebleed becomes an epitaxis, heavy periods a case of menorrhagia, a bruise an eccymosis, and a lousy head, a case of pediculosis capitis', comment Irish medical doctors Petr Skrabanek and James McCormick.[12]

In many cases, anatomical variants are invoked to explain psychosomatic problems. In this context Uwe Heyll remarks:

> This way, a kidney cyst will have to do as an explanation for a pain in the flank, minimal alterations of the spine's cervical vertebra are supposed to be the reason for headaches or dizziness attacks, a coincidentally found gallstone explains the pain in the upper abdomen, an uterus myoma causes lower abdominal pain, a floating kidney leads to problems during urination, a miniscule intestinal polyp explains digestion problems, or a slightly enlarged thyroid gland is claimed to be the cause of nervousness. Of course, none of the mentioned organ alterations has illness status. Nevertheless and owing to lack of better explanations, they are declared causes for the respective conditions.[13]

In particular, diagnoses for unexplainable phenomena should be chosen so as to be to the affected person's liking – at least this is what physicians from Edinburgh, Scotland recommend. In a study of eighty-six participants, they investigated people's reactions to different labels. When the doctor told them the disease was 'put on', 'hysterical', 'medically unexplained', 'psychosomatic' or 'stress-related', most people felt that they were not being taken seriously. The meaningless epithet 'functional', however, satisfied them. Therefore, the Scottish doctors 'call for the rehabilitation of "functional" as a useful and acceptable diagnosis for physical symptoms unexplained by disease'.[14]

The medical profession's code of honour requires diagnosing too. A doctor who correctly diagnoses a rare condition is greatly honoured; and one who gives a diagnosis where nothing is wrong commits a *faux pas*, but is considered cautious. An unforgivable mistake, however, is to overlook a true disease. Drs Petr Skrabanek and James McCormick have compared the effects of mistakes as follows:[15]

Type-1 mistake (no disease, but a diagnosis) and its consequences

1   A healthy person is declared a patient and exposed to unnecessary as well as risky follow-up examinations.
2   The affected person loses sight of his or her own health and is encouraged to slip into playing a sick-role.
3   The doctor is on the safe side, and avoids the risk of being sued for professional error; prosecution for 'superfluous diagnosis' is not to be feared.
4   Correction of type-1 mistake is unusual and difficult.

Type-2 mistake (disease, but no diagnosis given) and its consequences

1   The doctor is threatened by legal action and consequences because he or she overlooked a disease through negligence.
2   Medical colleagues will judge and ostracise the doctor for this mistake.
3   The doctor may be able, however, to correct the error (and thereby to disguise it), when illness progresses later on; the doctor may then produce an up-to-date version of the previously overlooked diagnosis.

Affected people might regard type-1 mistake as the most pleasant. Some healthy persons seem in fact to be longing for diagnosis, for it is a privilege: it entitles one to be sick and brings some advantages in life – for instance, early retirement. Personal well-being may increase as well, as soon as a diagnosis is given. A study compared 'positive' and 'negative' patient consultations. During the positive consultations, the test persons were given a clear diagnosis and the assurance that they would soon recover from the condition. In the negative consultations doctors explained to the patients that they were unable to tell them what was wrong with them. The result was that those people whom the doctor declared clearly ill were more content: 64 per cent of patients who had a positive consultation felt better afterwards. Among the patients who went through a negative consultation only 39 per cent felt better.

Non-diseases

With brazen audacity, ailments and epidemics that do not actually exist are invented: so-called non-diseases. In public, medical associations mostly deny the existence of non-diseases, leaving many practising doctors trying to figure out which of the many newly emerging clinical pictures are in some way justified and how they should deal with them.

Since the number of mock syndromes is on the rise and it is getting harder to make sense of the situation, the *British Medical Journal* has submitted questionnaires to its readership, consisting mainly of medics, to investigate what the twenty most common non-diseases are. To begin, the editors gave a definition for non-disease: 'a human process or problem that some have defined as a medical condition but where people may have better outcomes if the problem or process was not defined in that way'.

The doctors' imagination seemed to know no limits: almost 200 conditions were denoted as non-diseases. Some of them have already advanced into the official classification systems of medicine; others might still succeed.

Hit list of non-diseases[16]

1   Ageing
2   Work
3   Boredom
4   Bags under eyes
5   Ignorance
6   Baldness
7   Freckles
8   Big ears
9   Grey or white hair
10 Ugliness
11 Childbirth
12 Allergy to the twenty-first century
13 Jetlag
14 Unhappiness
15 Cellulite
16 Hangover
17 Anxiety about penis size/penis envy
18 Pregnancy
19 Road rage
20 Loneliness

Even more revealing than the list was the debate that subsequently flared up among journal readers. In hundreds of emails they disputed whether chronic fatigue syndrome, elevated cholesterol level, Oedipus complex, grieving, obesity, flatulence in babies or osteoporosis were in fact diseases or not. The medical laity can only watch in wonder at how divided the medical profession is with regard to the elementary question of which life processes and problems would be medically treatable at all. It is precisely this uneasy feeling – spiked with a good shot of scepticism – that Richard Smith, then chief editor of the *British Medical Journal*, sought to stir up. He says, 'Surely, everything is to be gained and nothing lost by raising consciousness about the slipperiness of the concept of disease.'

Therapies for caprices of nature

Everywhere in medicine, one comes across non-diseases. Children are often born slightly pigeon-toed, with their toes and forefoot turned in, a so-called sickle-foot. Many orthopaedists try to treat this whim of nature with massages, bandages and plaster; some even operate. However, the sickle-foot disappears on its own in 96 out of 100 children by the age of 3, as American researchers have found out. And even for the remaining 4 per cent, no foot problems in later life were detected.

The sickle-foot is not the only phenomenon which disappears over time, yet nevertheless provokes diligent treatment attempts. Some young people walk longer than their peers on knock-knees, which is normal in small children. This would put too much strain on the hip joints, speculated some physicians – and swiftly invented an impressive name for the alleged condition: 'prearthrotic deformation'. In the near future, this deformation would inevitably lead to arthrosis, a pathological alteration of the joint. In seeking prevention, doctors started, towards the end of the 1960s, to examine thigh bones of a whole generation by X-ray and if necessary to alter them through surgery. Through this procedure, the thigh was supposed to rest in a more advantageous position in relation to the hip joint. 'Some orthopaedists were almost possessed with the idea of surgery', remembers Lutz Jani of the Orthopaedic University Clinic in Mannheim, Germany.

Not until a decade after the beginning of this ghastly operating theatre episode were critical voices heard. At the end of the 1970s Jani published the sobering findings: prearthrotic deformation corrects itself completely in almost all cases. However, it took another decade until this knowledge kept the orthopaedists' operation frenzy in check.[17]

Among the favourite non-diseases in children were growing polyps and enlarged tonsils which were, in the past, surgically removed. In the year 1930, for example, 60 per cent of school children had had their tonsils removed by the age of 11, as a sample of 1,000 pupils in New York showed. The remaining 40 per cent were then examined as well – and doctors wanted to remove the tonsils of every other pupil. After another examination, only 65 pupils out of the initial 1,000 were considered healthy. A further examination of the children was not conducted, because there were no longer enough specialist doctors available.[18]

Since that time, the pool of alleged diseases has expanded to 40,000 variants, and every day new ones pop up. Thus, British researcher Tamara King questioned 530 women and immediately described a clinical picture named 'Shopping bulimia' (Shop 'til you drop).[19] Anyone who buys designer clothes and returns them to the shop after wearing them only once is supposed to be showing signs.

Diseases make a successful career

The English physician Thomas Sydenham (1624–89) assumed that a disease could be found and identified like a plant or animal species. In other words, diseases would occur in nature independently from the observer and would there be waiting to be discovered by the doctor. Reality is much less romantic. Diseases are often constructed; self-appointed experts decide their existence. How arbitrary the concept of disease is is revealed in the example of homosexuality. Psychiatrists regarded the affection for persons of the same sex as a medical condition that had to be treated. It was not until 1974 that members of the American Psychiatric Association decided by vote that from then on homosexuality should not be a disease any more. From one day to the next millions of people were thereby 'cured'. Some diseases are therefore not biological or psychological, but solely humanmade phenomena – and they may be born into the world in unlimited numbers.

The birth of a disease often starts with the fact that a doctor wants to have observed something anomalous. To begin with, only a few medical experts are convinced by the new syndrome. A manageable number of supporters meet at a conference, where a committee is appointed to publish a compendium that informs about the new syndrome and aims to raise interest. Now other doctors also become aware of the new phenomenon and start to search specifically for patients whose symptoms may fit. This selective perception could already cause a minor 'epidemic'. Many published papers and research reports then give the public the impression that doctors have discovered a new disease. The medical experts publish their findings in a specially established technical journal – critical reports are not included.

All that is left is the collecting of tell-tale signs which support the new condition. Falsification, the targeted search for counter-indications, is not attempted. The mutual assuring and confirming process leads finally among medical doctors and scientists to the fallacy that one had actually discovered a disease. The people who are suffering from the alleged syndrome are also pushing its expansion forward. They organise self-help groups and inform the public about their problem. The media present reports, whereupon the number of alleged patients increases further. In this phase, the burden of proof is upturned. Although the very existence of the syndrome is still to be doubted, its diagnosis and therapy have been established in the medical profession and in the public's perception as well.

This inventing of new conditions 'is an expression of doctors' efforts to find a suitable diagnosis for every patient', states Uwe Heyll from Düsseldorf, Germany. This way vague stomach aches would become a 'colon irritability', stress-related chest pain an 'effort syndrome', tiredness a 'chronic fatigue syndrome' and generalised aches and pains would turn into a mysterious rheumatism of the soft parts, named 'fibromyalgia'. Conversely to what the name (*fibra* – Latin for fibre, *myos* – Greek for muscle and *algos* – Greek for pain) might suggest, no noticeable alterations of muscles and tendons are detectable for this condition, which is almost solely observable in women.

A pill for every ill and an ill for every pill

Whether non-diseases grow into national epidemics is, to a considerable extent, up to the pharmaceutical industry. Only when a company has found a pill for a supposed condition is the latter systematically blown up into a threat. The 'pharmaceutical industry then becomes a key player in the process of medicalisation', comments London health expert David Gilbert. 'Once a drug is available, industry campaigns may seek to redefine the illness in the minds of doctors and of potential patients.' The alleged health problems would then be portrayed as a kind of illness that is primarily amenable to pharmaceutical treatment.[20]

Many people are very susceptible to this strategy. Whether a bald head, foul humour or corpulence, it's all the same – once modern medicine has served them a biological cause and the possibility of treatment for their problem, a bizarre transformation takes its course. The wish to be happier or the worry about losing one's hair is at once converted into a medical problem.

4 Risk factor merry-go-round

In most of the cases, when disease mongers want to label people as defective they do not feel their supposed defect at all. This applies particularly to measurable values like cholesterol level, blood pressure or bone density. These values change with age and influence the health condition of an individual in a way difficult to predict. It is true that lowering high blood pressure may reduce the risk of heart attack and stroke, but for most people the effect is minimal and health dealers sell new drugs for which an advantageous effect has not been proven at all.[1]

To do this, physicians' groups and pharmaceutical firms portray these risk factors as discrete diseases. Powerful and seemingly independent initiatives have emerged to take on this role; they are without exception sponsored by the industry. The limits they recommend are arbitrary and incompatible with the fluid transitions of biology. Such a way of thinking was criticised, centuries ago, by the great German writer Johann Wolfgang Goethe: 'Measuring a thing is a coarse act, which can only be applied to living bodies in a highly questionable manner.'

Most measured values are deemed risk factors, suspects medical doctor Uwe Heyll, only because they enable physicians to make a diagnosis in a convenient and seemingly objective way. Dr Heyll argues:

> We must ask ourselves why high blood pressure and cholesterol of all things have been recognised as medical risk factors. The answer is simple: because they are easy to measure. To determine blood pressure we only need an inflatable bag and a stethoscope, and verifying the cholesterol level is one of the easiest laboratory tests of all.[2]

The myth of bad cholesterol

A widespread pastime is occupying oneself with cholesterol levels. This is encouraged as much as possible by certain doctors and companies, which might profit from this multibillion business. Thus, the Federal Association of Practising Cardiologists, margarine producer Becel, pharmaceutical concern Pfizer and Roche Diagnostics enterprise regularly organise 'Health Initiatives', urging people to have their cholesterol levels tested. In a brochure displayed at pharmacies it says: 'Every person from the age of 30 onwards should know their cholesterol level and have it tested every other year.' According to the brochure, an elevated cholesterol level was 'one of the most significant risk factors' for heart and circulation diseases. The *Neue Apotheken Illustrierte* describes cholesterol as a 'health time bomb'.

None the less, the waxy substance is a vital element of the human body and is used in large quantities, for example in the brain: the thinking organ consists of 10 to 20 per cent cholesterol. Most body cells can produce it themselves, if supply is lacking through food intake. This is good news, because cells would die without the much-bemoaned molecule. In spite of this, for many people the mere mention of the word cholesterol brings premature death by cardiac arrest immediately to mind. For many it spoils their breakfast egg and their butter on toast, and fills them with uneasiness as they bite into their sausage. In 2001 alone, more than a million people in Germany, driven by conscience, had their cholesterol levels tested as part of the 'Health Initiative'. As expected, more than half of the tested persons had levels above the arbitrarily determined threshold of 5.2 millimoles or 200 milligrams.

The doctors and firms involved in the 'Health Initiative' are profiting directly: Roche Diagnostics is a producer of cholesterol-measuring equipment. Cardiologists, in turn, get more new patients to whom they preach about not eating butter, and so the margarine firm Becel benefits. At the end of the line there is Pfizer, which has a several billion turnover worldwide selling cholesterol-lowering drugs. Rarely has a medical campaign, which brands the majority of the people 'patients', been promoted by such a marketing extravaganza.

A committee from the American Heart Association even calls for regular cholesterol level tests in five-year-old children. Moreover, doctors should establish the risk of heart disease and the family smoking habits either before the child is born or immediately afterwards. Once the child is able to swallow solid food, goes the doctors' advice, the parents receive suggestions on how to provide their offspring with a diet low in cholesterol. Blood pressure should be controlled from their third birthday.[3]

Such early tests, however, do not allow one to draw conclusions about just how the tested child's health will develop. 'Screening children, even the 25 per cent with a family history of high blood cholesterol or early artery disease, is a waste of money that is likely to do more harm than good', argues Thomas B. Newman, epidemiologist from the University of California in San Francisco.[4]

If one were to take the preventive recommendations seriously, infants would have to be deprived of mother's milk – a true cholesterol bomb. In reality, it is breast-fed babies who thrive best, and no wonder, as the large amount of cholesterol from the mother's milk is needed for the growth of nerve cells and the brain.

The impression given by major national education programmes, namely that the cholesterol theory is proven knowledge, is deceiving. Many doctors have huge doubts as to whether cholesterol really plays such a villainous role in the drama of cardiac infarction. As early on as 1990, when the dubious threshold of 200 milligrams was propagated in Germany, experts like cardiologist Harald Klepzig from the German Heart Foundation in Frankfurt-upon-Main distanced themselves. He said at the height of the cholesterol hysteria:

> We would be happy if a single controlled medical study could be supplied which shows that human lives could be saved by lowering cholesterol. By contrast, it is not difficult to pick out ten studies showing that reducing fat is, rather, accompanied by a higher mortality.[5]

Paul Rosch, president of the American Institute of Stress and professor of medicine at the New Yorker Medical College, comments: 'The brain washing of the public has functioned so well that many people think that the lower their cholesterol level, the healthier they will be and the longer they would live. Nothing could be further from the truth.'[6]

In fact the claim that cholesterol is bad is not based on proof, but on just a few pieces of evidence – many of which do not withstand scrutiny. In 1953, researcher Ancel Keys from the University of Minnesota published a paper that would become the founding myth of the cholesterol theory. Keys showed a diagram which suggested a clear correlation between fat consumption and mortality through coronary heart diseases in six countries (Figure 1). 'The graph leaves barely any doubt about the correlation between food fat content and the

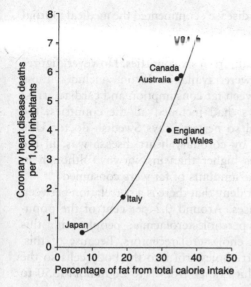

Figure 1 Coronary heart disease deaths in six countries
Source: Uffe Ravnskov with Udo Pollmer, *Mythos Cholesterin*, Stuttgart, 2002

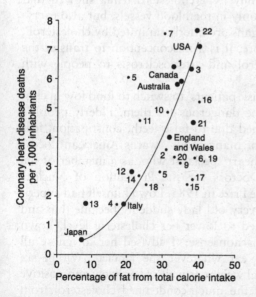

Figure 2 Coronary heart disease deaths in twenty-two countries
Source: Uffe Ravnskov with Udo Pollmer, *Mythos Cholesterin*, Stuttgart, 2002

risk of dying of coronary heart disease', commented the medical journal *Lancet* at the time.[7]

No matter how impressive the graph seems, it has a huge flaw. Keys took into consideration data from six countries. However, figures from twenty-two countries were available. If one includes these data, then the correlation between fat consumption and cardiac arrest disappears (Figure 2). If Keys 'had included all the countries, the graph would not have looked so perfect', says Swedish doctor Uffe Ravnskov. 'Mortality caused by coronary heart disease was, in the USA for example, three times higher than in Norway, although in both countries almost the same amounts of fat were consumed.'[8]

Critics like Ravnskov do not deny that there is a correlation between blood fat and coronary diseases. Around 0.2 per cent of the population are suffering from hypercholesterolaemia: people with this hereditary disease lack intact cholesterol receptors. Because of this, the blood can barely transport cholesterol into the body cells so the cholesterol level rises. The values range from 9 to 26 mmol/l (350 to 1,000 mg/dl). The affected persons do have a higher risk of dying from heart attack because they often become ill with a serious kind of arteriosclerosis. It is doubtful, though, whether this condition is comparable to the true arteriosclerosis. Autopsy studies of individuals who were suffering from family hypercholesterolaemia showed that cholesterol accumulated not only in the blood vessels, but also everywhere in the body. 'Many organs are utterly saturated by cholesterol', says Uffe Ravnskov. Therefore, it is a misconception to transfer the correlation between cholesterol and arteriosclerosis to people with normal cholesterol levels.

When doctors urge older 'risk patients' to switch to food low in cholesterol, it could even become dangerous for them. Elderly people's nutrition is 'already diminished due to false teeth, constipation, loss of appetite and intolerance of many foods', warns American doctor Bernard Lown, a renowned heart specialist who, as a member of the organisation International Doctors for the Prevention of Nuclear War, received the Nobel Peace Prize in 1985. Lown himself had experience, as a doctor, of how a very old lady suddenly became thin and declined because she had tried to lower her cholesterol level. Lown put an end to this dangerous nonsense: 'I advised her to ignore all that medical advice and to eat whatever she fancied. Within six months she regained her initial weight as well as her lively and positive mood.'[9] In reality, we need the much-condemned cholesterol from infancy to old age.

The statin saga

The so-called statins inhibit the manufacture of mevalonic acid, which is needed for the synthesis of cholesterol. As a result, body cells primarily use cholesterol from food intake, which lowers its level in the blood. This quality – for the pharmaceutical industry – turns statins into the ultimate drug. The target group is enormous: namely that majority of the population whose cholesterol level was previously defined as elevated and therefore as requiring treatment. Since these people are otherwise in good health, they live long enough to swallow statins over decades, on a daily basis. Actually, these cholesterol inhibitors have proven to be real money machines on the pharmaceutical market, particularly because they enjoyed the benefit of patent protection and were sold at high prices (around one to two Euros per daily ration). The Pfizer enterprise is about to achieve a yearly turnover of $10 billion with its statin called Lipitor – it is already the biggest pharmaceutical bestseller of all time. Its competitor Zocor from Merck makes a marginally less impressive profit of $7.5 billion. In the United States 5.4 per cent of the adult population are taking statins; in the whole world, there are 44 million consumers.

In the summer of 2002, findings from a strictly controlled study that included more than 20,500 people over a period of five years showed not only that this medicine is expensive, but also that it has a measurable benefit. According to the Heart Protection Study conducted in Great Britain, the frequency of blood vessel diseases and their consequences, such as cardiac infarct, stroke and amputations, may be lowered by 24 per cent through a daily intake of 40 milligrams of the statin Zocor. The number of deaths decreased, from 14.7 to 12.9 per cent, compared with a control group that was not given a statin drug.

This means, in absolute figures, that if 1,000 people, who are at risk of developing a vascular disease, take the statin daily over a five-year period, then 70 to 100 may avoid having to have an operation on their vascular system. The number of deaths might be lowered by 25. If 10 million risk patients were treated, 50,000 deaths from vascular diseases might be avoided. Since a daily dosage of 40 milligrams of statin costs around two Euros, this would cost the health system 7 billion Euros.[10]

However, as the Heart Protection Study revealed, cholesterol is not a risk factor at all, for even people with low cholesterol levels benefited from the daily statin intake. In other words, it is not the lowering of cholesterol that provides a protective effect: the statins seem to work in a rather different way, probably by stabilising the vascular walls and inhibiting inflammations. In view of these surprising findings, measuring cholesterol levels seems even more pointless than ever. Charles George, medical director of the British Heart Foundation, suggests: 'The unambiguous message of the study is: treat risks, not cholesterol levels!'

Screening for high blood pressure

Measuring blood pressure is probably the most common procedure in medicine – and the most common reason for instigating long-term medical treatment of healthy people. The procedure seems innocuous enough, quite painless and lasts no longer than two minutes: the pressure that the heart exerts in pumping blood through the body is measured with an inflatable bag, attached around the upper arm. The heart's pressure is not constant. It reaches its highest value when the left ventricle contracts and pumps blood into the circulation. At this moment, the systolic blood pressure is measured. The thus-created pressure wave keeps the blood flowing as the heart relaxes and the pressure comes to its lowest point, the diastolic blood pressure. The values are measured in 'mm Hg' (this means millimetre of mercury column).

It is true that high blood pressure is considered one of the most important risk factors for the development of abnormal arterial hardening (arteriosclerosis) and its consequences, such as cardiac infarct, stroke and kidney failure. However, it is medically controversial from which value onwards the affected person should be treated. At the beginning of the 1990s in Germany, values of 160 over 100 were considered in need of treatment. Therefore, the whole Federal Republic counted around 7 million hypertensive people. Then, the German League for the Fight against High Blood Pressure, an interest group founded in 1974 consisting of physicians and pharmaceutical companies' employees, recommended a new threshold – 140 over 90 – and overnight the number of affected people tripled. This private organisation single-handedly turned high blood pressure into a national disease.[11] Twenty of its members, who are without exception employees of pharmaceutical companies, serve the League as 'patronising members of the board of trustees'.[12] League spokesman Eckhart Böttcher-Bühler announced: 'Pharmaceutical companies buy brochures from us and their travelling reps distribute them among the public.'

In more than 90 per cent of all cases, doctors do not find any cause for the alleged 'high' blood pressure values; they then talk about an

'essential' or 'primary' hypertension, which camouflages their ignorance and sounds good to the patients. Although the inexplicable phenomenon — it it is even worth calling it that — is for the affected
person only a risk factor, it has been elevated to the status of a disease
in its own right by physicians and pharmaceutical firms. In the
League's patients' magazine *Druckpunkt*, for instance, it says:

> High blood pressure is called essential or primary if it occurs as a
> distinct clinical picture and not only as a consequence or symptom
> of another disease. The elevation of the blood pressure is therefore
> the essential characteristic of this disease.[13]

Many people get ill just by looking at a doctor in a white coat – the
experience makes their blood pressure rise. In a trial with 200 patients
from three family doctors' practices, English physicians confirmed that
this 'white coat effect' is very common and could lead to a number of
wrong diagnoses. During the trial, either the patients measured their
own blood pressure or it was measured for them, either by a practice
nurse or by a doctor. As was shown, the respect-inspiring figure of
the doctor pushed the blood pressure highest. The values measured
by doctors were an average of 18.9 mm HG higher than other
measurements. Were doctors to rely solely on blood pressure values
they had measured themselves, a large number of patients would in
fact be treated unnecessarily. The authors of the study demand: 'It is
time to stop using high blood pressure readings documented by general
practitioners to make treatment decisions.'[14]

The fact that people with medium severe and severe hypertension
have to be treated with blood pressure lowering drugs is not open for
discussion among physicians. These real hypertension patients were,
'however, only a small part of the total number of hypertensive
people', argues Dr Heyll from Düsseldorf. The vast majority of
affected patients are in fact 'hypertensive healthy' people: their blood
pressure readings were only slightly above average, and they are otherwise healthy. Yet, most doctors would urge these people also to be
treated with blood pressure lowering drugs, even though there are
no scientific grounds for this therapy and the tablets could have
unpleasant side effects. Uwe Heyll sums up: 'The drug treatment of
mild blood pressure is an overuse of therapy, which might be more
damaging than beneficial for most of the affected people.'[15]

Anxiety spreading bone lobby

The age of human beings can be detected from their bones. At the age of 35, the skeleton reaches its maximal density. During the following years bone mass reduces. More of it is lost than is rebuilt. This process, which consumes 1 to 1.5 per cent of bone density per year, affects the spinal column first. When somebody celebrates their seventieth birthday, they have lost approximately one-third of their bone substance – and, by the way, one-third of muscle mass too.

This bone atrophy is therefore a natural, though unpleasant, accompanying phenomenon of ageing. Most elderly people do not feel specific restrictions; however, for some elderly people, bones become so porous and brittle that they cannot withstand certain strain any longer. Vertebrae might break, leading to an extremely bent back. Although men are affected as well, the condition is commonly called 'widow's hump'. In addition, porous and brittle bones are partially to blame for frequent fractures of the arm or the neck of the femur in elderly people (75 years plus). In Strasbourg teaching pathologist Jean-Frédéric Lobstein (1777–1835) gave the age-related condition its name: osteoporosis ('brittle bones').

For decades to come, the term osteoporosis would be used only when the lessening of bone mass had actually led to a fracture. Based on information from the Federal Statistics Office, the diagnosis 'fracture of the neck of the femur' was given in Germany in 1995 in 74,803 cases in persons over 74 years of age. This is equivalent to a relative percentage of 1.2 for this age group.

This figure, which probably corresponds to figures in other industrial nations, does not warrant the label 'national disease' – and so osteoporosis has been completely reinvented at the instigation of pharmaceutical companies. The foundation stone for this was laid in 1940 when American physician Fuller Albright (1900–69) announced that one type of osteoporosis in women was caused by hormone deficiency and could therefore be treated with oestrogen: the industry's interest was aroused.

The American oestrogen producer Ayerst Laboratories sponsored, in 1982, a nationwide campaign in the United States to spread the word that osteoporosis was a threat to menopausal women. Until then, only very few women, not only in the United States but also worldwide, had ever heard the word 'osteoporosis'. Numerous programmes on radio and TV as well as magazine articles and advertisements transformed this state of affairs. Fifteen years on, 'Premarin', an oestrogen preparation from the firm of Ayerst, is the most frequently administered prescription drug in the United States.

Researchers Marianne Whatley and Nancy Worcester from the University of Wisconsin, Madison analysed the pharmaceutical campaign and explained its success by the fact that it specifically played on women's fears. The information, for example about fracture of the neck of the femur, Whatley and Worcester said, was compiled in a way that induced fear.

> For example, a popular guide to preventing osteoporosis states: 'The consequences of hip fractures can be devastating. Less than one-half of all women who suffer a hip fracture regain normal function. 15 per cent die shortly after their injury, and nearly 30 per cent die within a year.' The fear for women is that even if they survive a hip fracture, they may face long years of dependency and immobility.[16]

Not only Ayerst Laboratories, but also other enterprises have thrived as a result of such marketing strategies. Between 1980 and 1986, the turnover of calcium preparations rose dramatically. A brand of diet-cola with added calcium was able to triple its sales on some markets.

However, to elevate osteoporosis to the rank of a mass phenomenon did require an official redefinition of the disease. In 1993, the Rorer Foundation, along with the two companies Sandoz Pharmaceuticals and SmithKlineBeecham, sponsored a World Health Organisation (WHO) meeting where exactly this step was taken. Even 'gradual decline in bone mass with age' was, according to the WHO, to be regarded as osteoporosis.[17] Since then, the pharmaceutical industry, a German physician argues, has the chance 'to provide half of the population of forty and over with medicaments until old age'.[18]

In order to diagnose the new condition, a cunning bone density measure has been devised. Most of the time, X-rays are used. The denser the bone, the more the X-rays are toned down. This is then analysed by computer and the results compared with the bone density of a healthy 35-year-old person. The procedure establishes a diminished bone density in nearly every older person – precisely because bone decline is as much part of ageing as, for example, getting wrinkles.

To describe this process, nevertheless, as pathological, the WHO had to lay down arbitrary limits. Accordingly, osteoporosis is diagnosed if bone mass is approximately 20 to 35 per cent below the normal value – or more than 2.5 standard deviation (SD) below the norm. A SD value of 1 to 2.5 below the norm is regarded as 'osteopenia'– a type of preliminary stage of bone atrophy.

By this definition, the WHO has expanded the clinical picture of osteoporosis dramatically. Nowadays, it is no longer a broken bone, but rather too much decline in bone mass that labels a person a patient, and requires them to swallow the industry's calcium preparations and other medicines. Even a slightly diminished bone mass is depicted as something threatening: as osteopenia.

At the behest of the WHO whole sections of the population suddenly fell ill in 1993: 31 per cent of women between 70 and 79 have since suffered from osteoporosis; as far as women over 80 are concerned, 36 per cent are regarded sick – even if they've never broken a bone in their whole life.

The bone lobby accepted the WHO's guidelines with more than gratitude. 'Osteoporosis is a disease!' writes Dr Klaus Peter from the University of Munich in a brochure for World Osteoporosis Day, October 2002, and warns also: 'Men shouldn't allow themselves to be lulled into a false sense of security.' The conference in Munich (the patron was the Bavarian prime minister's wife Karin Stoiber) was sponsored by pharmaceutical companies that offer preparations against osteoporosis.[19] The WHO's definition grants the enterprises huge turnovers. Every other woman over 45 whose bone density measurement indicates osteoporosis opts, within six months, for treatment with appropriate recommended preparations.

The WHO experts failed to give a scientific justification for their decision. When the German Federal Committee of Physicians and Health Insurers inquired of the WHO, as to the study results the decision was based on, the competent official would or could not quote any sources.[20]

No wonder: the benefit of bone density measurements in pain-free patients is not proven. German, American and Swedish studies – independently of one another – drew this conclusion. Experts from the Office of Health Technology Assessment from the University of British Columbia in Vancouver, Canada, have presented a 174-page report on the question of whether diagnosing gives any benefit at all. Their result is also unambiguous: 'Research evidence does not support [either whole population or selective] bone mineral density testing of well women at or near menopause as a means to predict future fractures.'[21]

Bone density measuring has recently been deleted from the service catalogue of statutory health insurers in Germany. This has not quelled physicians' zeal: nowadays they are hoping that elderly people might fork out for the useless diagnosis themselves. And so, they are selling the bone mineral density test on the 'individual health service' (HIS), for which patients pay from their own pockets. 'Doctors, who want to own HIS in their practice, need a high [life] of [............] in their "potential buyers" and the right situation', is the guidance offered by the *Münchener Medizinische Wochenschrift* to its readers from the medical profession. The opportunity would often arise in conversation: 'A menopausal lady with her osteoporosis worries will probably be grateful for her doctor's suggestion of osteoporosis diagnosis and prophylaxis.'[22]

Health – 100 per cent metabolic disease

Researchers claim to have detected nearly 300 influences and habits which are risk factors of coronary heart diseases alone, so the Irish physicians Skrabanek and McCormick mockingly reveal. Medical experts count among the sources of danger elevated cholesterol levels, high blood pressure, smoking, obesity, diabetes, low HDL cholesterol level, high LDL cholesterol level, selenium, alcohol, poor exercise habits, not having after-lunch naps, too little fish, living in Scotland, having English as one's mother tongue, suffering from severe phobias, being too punctual, not taking fish liver oil and snoring.[23]

So what exactly would a man who does not have to fear cardiac arrest in this risk-strewn world actually look like?

G. S. Myers paints for us the following picture: he would be

> an effeminate embalmer completely lacking in physical or mental alertness and without drive, ambition, or competitive spirit, who has never attempted to meet a deadline of any kind; a man with poor appetite, subsisting on fruits and vegetables laced with corn and whale oil, detesting tobacco, spurning ownership of radio, television, or motorcar, with full head of hair but scrawny and unathletic appearance, yet constantly straining his puny muscles by exercise. Low in income, blood pressure, blood sugar, uric acid, and cholesterol, he has taken nicotinic acid, pyridoxine, and long-term anti-coagulant therapy ever since his prophylactic castration.

A woman with low risk of heart attack would be: 'a bicycling, unemployed, hypo-beta-lipoproteinaemic, hypolipemic, underweight, premenopausal female dwarf living in a crowded room on the island of

Crete before 1925 and subsisting on a diet of uncoated cereals, safflower oil and water'.[24]

The list of alleged risk factors is getting longer every day – and each entry more incredible. Women, for example, should have early pregnancies to avoid breast cancer. In order to combat cancer of the womb, however, they should remain virgins. Childless women, on the other hand, are at higher risk of developing cancer of the large intestine. Preventive medicine has just become so out of hand that nobody can live up to it any more.

5 Insanity as the norm

> Do you know what you need?
> One gram of soma.
>
> Aldous Huxley, *Brave New World*

What is the difference between sanity and insanity? David Rosenhan, psychologist at Stanford University, California, tried to answer this question in a self-trial in 1968: the researcher, at the time 40 years old, did not wash himself for several days. He also abstained from brushing his teeth. Instead of shaving, he allowed his beard to sprout and he wore dirty clothes. Under a false name he then arranged an appointment at a psychiatric institution. His wife dropped him off at the front entrance.

At the reception, Rosenhan told the doctors about voices he claimed to have heard. These, he said, he could barely understand, but had said 'empty', 'hollow' and 'thud'. What the psychiatrists did not know was that he was pretending to have precisely these symptoms because in all the literature Rosenhan hadn't found a single psychosis that would have matched his supposed symptoms. From the moment of his admission, however, the researcher went back to completely normal behaviour. He talked to other patients and to staff – and waited.

During the following years, the trial was repeated several times. Rosenhan and seven sane 'comrades-in-arms' were admitted under false names and with the same symptoms into twelve mental hospitals. According to the rules of the experiment, the pseudo-patients were supposed to get out of the institutions entirely by themselves. Therefore, they behaved completely normally and helpfully; they obeyed the rules inside the institutions and took the prescribed psycho-pharmaceuticals – or at least pretended to do so. Before the admission, they had practised putting tablets under their tongue instead of swallowing them.

In every trial the question was: how long would it take the psychiatrists to discover the fake patient and throw him out of the clinic on his ear? The result: none of the phoney patients was ever discovered; they were kept inside for three weeks on average and then all discharged with a psychiatric diagnosis, most of the time 'schizophrenia in remission'.

The fake patients, between them, received 2,100 tablets. They included all kinds of different preparations – although all of them had displayed the same symptoms. In one of the institutions, Rosenhan was kept for a record fifty-two days. 'This was a very long time', he remembers, 'but in the end, I almost got used to the hospital routine.'[1]

By 'cross-checking' the first experiment, David Rosenhan made a mockery of the psychiatric establishment for a second time. He announced to the doctors of a mental hospital that he would infiltrate the clinic with fake patients in the coming three months. Only, in reality, he did not send them sane people at all, but 193 real patients for admission. Nevertheless, 10 per cent of the psychologically troubled individuals were dismissed from the institution – on the grounds that they were sane.

The 1973 publication of these trials in *Science* ('On being sane in insane places') shook the credibility of psychiatry. The self-trials revealed the arbitrariness of psychiatrists' judgements. Based on what criteria do they determine the boundaries between mentally healthy and ill? Psychologist Rosenhan provided an answer that gives much cause for thought: 'However much we may be personally convinced that we can tell the normal from the abnormal, the evidence is simply not compelling.'[2]

The new illnesses of the mind

This dilemma has not quelled the psychiatrists' zeal (or should we call it an occupational hazard?) for reinterpreting normal conduct and turning it into treatment-requiring behaviour. Rather the opposite is the case: the number of mental illnesses in the official 'classification systems' has seen a curious increase in recent years. In the catalogue of the American veterans' administration after the Second World War, just 26 disorders were listed. The currently *Diagnostic and Statistical Manual of Mental Disorders* (DSM-IV) from the Association of American Psychiatrists includes 395 distinct illnesses that can be diagnosed and consequently accounted for. The WHO's *International*

Classification of Diseases (ICD-10), customary in Europe, is similar to the American list and has also been enriched by a multitude of disorders.

The epidemic-like spread of delusion and insanity not only provides the tiers of psychiatrists and psychotherapists with their bread and butter salaries, but also grants pharmaceutical companies brilliant business balance sheets. Sell an illness in order to sell medications – this strategy is particularly typical for psychiatry, precisely due to its nature. The diagnostic criteria that it operates with are especially fluid. The enlightening campaigns of the pharmaceutical industry target mild mental conditions, which might apply to a wide circle of people. Rebellious children, for example, are certified as having the disorder 'infantile oppositional defiance behaviour'.

In industrialised countries, financial connections particularly between psychiatrists and pharmaceutical companies are the norm. The German Society for Psychiatry, Psychotherapy and Mental Health, for example, accepts for its activity 'support' from the enterprises Astra Zeneca, Aventis Pharmaceutical Deutschland, Lilly, Novartis Pharmaceutical and Organon. 'Press releases' sponsored by these companies draw the public's attention to ever-new psychological troubles. Thus the September 2002 issue reads: 'Depressions, anxiety disorders, and addictions – these are the new diseases of civilisation.'[3]

Some experts find this strange. British psychiatrist David Healy notes:

> The techniques used to market information have developed to the point where significant changes in the mentality of both clinicians and the public can be produced within a matter of few years. Increases in the incidence of conditions by a thousandfold do not appear to surprise clinicians.[4]

For patients, clinicians and pharmaceutical firms, the disease catalogues are of immense importance. Only if a condition is listed do health insurers pay the costs for medicaments and therapy. Since 'premenstrual syndrome' was included in the US hit-list of mental illnesses, psychiatrists too are now able to treat the alleged female disorder – if necessary with psycho-pharmaceuticals. For this market, the firm Lilly has recycled a well-known product. Since the patent for bestseller pill Prozac has expired, the company now markets the same substance under the name 'Sarafem', as a pill for premenstrual dysphoric disorder (PMDD). Thus, psychiatrists are competing with gynaecologists – giving hormone preparations a shot to treat the same phenomenon.

Interestingly, the antidepressant drug's licence for PMDD was withdrawn in 2003. A committee of the European Agency for the Evaluation of Medicinal Products (Emea) in London concluded that, 'PMDD is not a well-established disease entity across Europe'. And indeed, a few months later the drug manufacturer Eli Lilly informed health professionals in a letter that it had removed premenstrual dysphoric disorder from the list of indications – one invented illness less.[5]

Many of the 'new complaints of the psyche', as Basle psychiatrist Asmus Finzen calls them, are however nothing more than the expression of normal life's ups and downs. The desire for solitude is blown up into an 'antisocial personality', and grief, in turn, finds its way into psychology – as pathological 'adjustment disorder' (ICD-10, F43). The latter is supposed to designate various 'states of subjective complaints and emotional impairments, which affect social functioning and achievement; they occur during the adjustment process after a decisive life-change, a distressing life-event, or severe physical illness'.

Psychiatrist Finzen has quantified the spread of mental illnesses according to the catalogue DSM-IV. His findings: 58 per cent of the population suffer at one time or another from a personality disorder – it is therefore *normal* to be mentally ill.[6]

For the armies of alleged psychiatric patients the industry has a manifold supply of medicaments in store. Antidepressants, especially the selective serotonin reuptake inhibitors (SSRI), of which Prozac is the first and best known example, have become fashion drugs for gloominess, sadness and anxiety. The green and white Prozac capsules increase the amount of serotonin in the brain and so raise the mood. Serotonin is an important messenger agent in the brain; it affects feelings like pride and self-esteem. It is true that SSRI have side effects like diminished sexual drive and in rare cases an increased disposition to violence and suicide. Nevertheless, many people who take SSRI say that the substance makes them more clear headed, self-confident and extrovert. Therefore, it has paved the way for a 'cosmetic psychiatry', as American psychiatrist and author Peter D. Kramer put it in his bestseller *Listening to Prozac*. People who were not ill in the first place were taking Prozac to feel 'better than good'. The former service providers for mentally ill people are now running a health industry of mental happiness.

One side effect of the mood enhancers reaches particularly far: since it has become clear that SSRI and other pharmaceuticals modify certain facets of human behaviour, these traits and moods are being systematically medicalised. 'Anxiety' in particular has aroused drug manufacturers' greed. At the beginning of 2001, twenty-seven different substances worked their way through the development pipelines of the industry, all of which were supposed to be marketed as remedies for ᴀₙₓᵢₑₜᵧ ᵈᵢₛₒᵣᵈₑᵣ.[7] ᴛₕᵢₛ ᵣₑₛₑₘᵦₗₑₛ ᵃ ₚᵣₑᵈᵢᶜₜᵢₒₙ ᵒᶠ ₜₕₑ ᵦᵣₐᵥₑ ₙₑw World that Aldous Huxley painted. In his novel, 2,000 pharmacologists and biochemists are entrusted with the development of a popular drug that makes people happy and uncritical. With 'soma', one can 'take a holiday from reality whenever one wants'.[8]

SSRI initially used for the treatment of severe depressions are, in western countries, prescribed as remedies for a colourful medley of disorders, which did not even exist a few years ago. The drug Paroxetine, for example, is licensed in the United States now for generalised anxiety disorder, panic disorder, compulsive disorder and post-traumatic stress disorder.

With a million dollar budget to spend, seemingly obscure phenomena are propagated to tap into a new and constant stream of clientele. American consumer protector Arthur Levin says: 'The symptomatology is so broad and vague that almost any of us could say, yeah, that is me!'[9] Disorders akin to already acknowledged diseases are cunningly invented. In the orbit of depression, clinicians and industry claim to have identified a condition, which they call 'dysthymia'.

'Tired, despondent, full of self-doubt – who among us can say they never had phases when the whole world seemed all doom and gloom?' asks the German Society for Psychiatry, Psychotherapy and Mental Health. It claims that up to 3.3 million Germans experienced negative emotions as a constant state yet these emotions 'are not recognised as a clinical picture often enough and treated accordingly'.[10] In the vernacular, the dysthymia patient is called by the usual name: misery guts.

Another example of the procreation of disorders: 'post-traumatic stress disorder' has recently had a daughter named 'acute stress disorder'. According to psychiatrists, post-traumatic stress disorder can occur in 10 to 30 per cent of people who are personally involved in traumatic events like war or kidnapping. Meanwhile, however, some people who experience such events only from the comfort of their TV settee become patients too: they become ill with 'acute stress disorder', a condition that allegedly requires treatment and has recently made it into the diagnoses catalogue DSM-IV.

In children psychiatric disorders are also multiplying: since it has become a known fact that certain substances alter certain modes of behaviour in children, precisely these modes of behaviour are depicted as pathological and requiring treatment – consequently, they take a psycho pill with their break-time snack (see Chapter 6).

Diagnosis: unsociable

The story of shyness reveals which mechanisms are set in motion
to establish a new disease on the market: in 1998 the company
SmithKline Beecham applied to the US agency FDA to license the use
of the drug 'Paxil' as a remedy for a phenomenon that would be
called 'social phobia' and later on 'social anxiety disorder' (SAD).
This meant an allegedly diagnosable form of unsociability or shyness.
In 1980, it was included in the American DSM and classified as
'extremely rare'.

Nevertheless, the syndrome seemed suitable for expansion. Whose
heart does not beat faster if they have to deliver a speech? Who does
not suffer from stage fright? In surveys, around 50 per cent of people
describe themselves as rather shy.

During the ongoing licensing procedure, the pharmaceutical company started to publicise the illness potential of shyness. To 'position
social anxiety disorder as a severe condition', as the trade journal
PR News put it, the company engaged the New York based public
relations firm Cohn & Wolfe. Soon afterwards, the firm invented a
slogan alluding to the possibility of having an allergic reaction to
others around them: 'Imagine Being Allergic to People'.

American bus shelters were wallpapered with advertisement posters
of a dejected-looking young man: 'You blush, sweat, shake – even
find it hard to breathe. That's what social anxiety disorder feels like.'
The posters made no reference to psycho pills or pharmaceutical
companies. What they referred to instead was a 'social anxiety disorder coalition' consisting of three apparently non-profit groups: the
American Psychiatric Association, the Anxiety Disorders Association
of America and the patient group Freedom from Fear.

However, the seemingly charitable parties did not come together by
coincidence: the coalition received financial support from SmithKline
Beecham.[11] And it was on the instructions of this coalition that PR
firm Cohn & Wolf answered the media's inquiries. The firm issued a
video press release and distributed a statement saying that SAD 'affects
up to 13.3 per cent of the population'. SAD was thereby the third most
frequent psychiatric illness in the United States, right after depression
and alcoholism.

Yet psychiatrists had previously consistently stated that only 2 to
3 per cent of the population were battling with this problem. How
then did this bizarre increase of shy people come about? The million-
fold expansion of pathological shyness happened as a result of a
decision taken by just a few on a psychiatrists' committee – it altered

the definition of social anxiety disorder. On the one hand, the scientists included a general subtype of the disorder (generalised anxiety disorder or GAD) in the clinical picture; on the other hand, they cancelled a strict diagnostic criterion, namely the 'compulsory desire to avoid'. Since then, shy persons can already be diagnosed as ill, if their timidity causes them 'definite difficulties'.[12]

'To put a face on the disorder', Cohn & Wolf swiftly provided journalists with eloquent patients. 'Everything took 10 times more effort for me than it did for anyone else', one woman told the *Chicago Tribune*. 'The thing about GAD is that worry can be a full-time job. So if you add that up with what I was doing, which was being a full-time achiever, I was exhausted, constantly exhausted.'[13] A woman by the name of Grace Dailey who also appeared in a marketing video was often quoted. Psychiatrist Jack Gorman, who obviously did not act from selfless motives, was seen too.[14] According to inquiries from the British *Guardian*, the man rendered his services to SmithKline Beecham and at least twelve other pharmaceutical companies as a paid consultant.

The campaign for social anxiety disorder has led to a measurable success. During the two years before the licensing of Paxil, fewer than fifty contributions on the subject were publicised in the US mass media. But in mid May 1999, when the FDA announced its decision regarding the licensing of Paxil, hundreds of newspaper and TV reports emerged. By the end of 2001, Paxil, the remedy for generalised and social anxiety disorder had advanced into the top group of anti-depressants in a head-to-head with the now classic Prozac.

In Germany too, anxiety disorder has set in, according to researchers from Dresden. In a questionnaire survey among 20,000 patients who went to their GP, 5.3 per cent, so they claim, were suffering from generalised anxiety disorder and one in four of the questioned citizens had singular symptoms of the disorder. The result promises a lot of work for the sponsor of the survey – the 'think positive firm' Wyeth.[15]

'The rather widespread assumption that modern civilisation engendered the emergence of mental illnesses, cannot be proven in a strictly scientific sense', the *Brockhaus-Lexikon* realised as early as 1892. In the twentieth century, the number of mentally ill people in society remained constant, says Basle psychiatrist Asmus Finzen. Two per thousand have a severe psychological illness; 2 per cent are in psychiatric treatment; and approximately 20 to 30 per cent of the population are at any given time in 'poor mental health'. However, these personal problems are often short-lived and disappear on their own, argues Finzen: Someone who is feeling out of sorts today, might be in good spirits again tomorrow.[16]

6 Psycho pill with break-time snack

The small white tablets alter children. In the past, Nina, an eight-year-old primary school pupil from Mittelehrenbach in Franconia, used to fidget. It took her three hours to do her homework and she would always tell her mother: 'I've got so many things in my head.'

One and a half years ago, however, things changed. Nina started taking daily 'concentration pills', as the family calls them. 'She can cope better in school and works more conscientiously', Nina's mother says, while her daughter plays a children's tune on the recorder. For a long time she hesitated to give her daughter the medication. But without Ritalin, things did not work: 'It's just that Nina wants to function normally.'

Felix, a fair-haired nine-year-old from near Forchheim has changed too, and – from his parents' point of view – for the better. In the past, the son was 'restless, constantly moving and couldn't concentrate', the mother says, 'there was something wrong with the child.' She doesn't think that's the case any more. Since Felix has been taking his daily dose of Ritalin, he has been more approachable. 'He can also sit down and read a book.' In primary school, things were much better. In dictation, Felix achieved a 'C plus' today. The mother beams: 'Ritalin really is a miracle remedy.'[1]

Like Nina and Felix, more than 50,000 children in Germany take daily doses of psycho-stimulants that are supposed to make them calm and attentive. The pills are meant to fight a condition that seems to be spreading in epidemic proportions: the attention deficit disorder (ADD), which is often said to be accompanied by 'hyperactivity' (ADHD).

With the increasing number of diagnoses, the number of diminutive consumers is also increasing. Ritalin and Medikinet, the names of two competing ADHD medicaments, are selling better than ever before. Use of the active agent methylphenidate, which falls under the narcotics law, has risen sharply in the recent past, so the experts at Federal Opium Bureau in Bonn tell us. The stimulant affects the brain directly and increases attention. In 1993, only 44 kilograms of methylphenidate was consumed, but by 2001, this figure had already risen to 693 kilograms – in only one decade a twenty-fold increase.

Much larger than the quantity of prescriptions is the number of parents who fear that their offspring are suffering from the fateful disease. There are more than sixty books in German on the subject of ADHD to quench the thirst for information. Hundreds of people attend events to become members of the attentive audiences when psychologists, clinicians and affected persons discuss the most important questions involved: How do I know if my child is affected? What is to blame, the parents' upbringing or the genes? Can Ritalin help? And is ADHD even a disease at all – or is it just a fashion craze?

As always when upbringing and children's welfare are involved, the debate is passionate and rife with accusations. People who give their child the psycho pill with their break-time snack are quickly judged uncaring parents; the ones who pronounce themselves against Ritalin are quickly accused of being friends with the Scientologists. (This sect condemns any psycho drug as devil's stuff, only to propagate their own beliefs as the key to a better life.)

Horror stories about the misuse of methylphenidate inflame feelings even further. In the United States, youths and young adults are consuming the children's pill as a lifestyle drug to control hunger and fight off tiredness. The tablets are swallowed or crushed into a powder and sniffed. 'The abuse of this substance has been documented among narcotic addicts who dissolve the tablets in water and inject the mixture', the US Ministry of Justice says. The injections might cause 'serious damage to the lungs and retina of the eye', the authority warns, as well as 'severe psychological addiction'.

As in the United States where approximately 5 million pupils take methylphenidate day in and day out, in Germany too, no other mental disorder in children and adolescents is diagnosed more frequently than ADHD. According to estimates, between 2 and 10 per cent of all children are supposed to be affected – statistically, that equates to around two fidgety children per class in need of medical help.

The ADHD hysteria seems unstoppable. Not only are doctors looking for undiscovered cases, but teachers too are screening their classes. In Hamburg schools, for example, leaflets ('Help for Self-Help') are circulated to sharpen the teaching staff's eyes for affected children. In Felix's case, it was also the class teacher who insisted on a medical examination. Soon afterwards, the boy started to receive the 'dope', as methylphenidate is called by some parents in the Franconian town.

Elsewhere, mothers text or call their children on the mobile, just to remind them to take their tablets next break. Sometimes, the teachers even hand out the pills – legally tricky, since they are dealing with a narcotic. Older pupils carry pillboxes that emit a sound signal when the next dose is due.

Recently, a growing number of adults too have been gripped by pathological distraction and unrest. 'Hyperactivity is not a children's disease', the German Society for Psychiatry, Psychotherapy and Mental Health claims. On federal German soil, 'up to 2 million adults' suffered from similar symptoms. 'Concentration deficiencies and undisciplined impulsiveness make it difficult for them to cope with everyday life.' Psycho pills are supposed to put things right: it was 'shown that adults, just like children, respond well to stimulating medicaments'.[2]

The industry already has its new target group by the scruff of its neck. 'ADHD, a life-long loyal companion', rejoices Ritalin producer, the global concern Novartis.[3] In May 2002, it invited physicians to Basle to instruct them in how the condition can be treated with 'stimulants and/or antidepressants'.

But Novartis cares most of all about our children. The concern has recently launched a picture book for the little ones. The pharma-tale tells the story of the octopus 'Hippihopp' who gets 'terribly scolded' because he is 'everywhere and nowhere' and prone to accidents and mishaps. But fortunately, the turtle doctor knows what Hippihopp has: 'an attention-deficit syndrome!' Moreover, it knows what Hippi's lacking: 'a small white tablet'.

Behind the rampant drug consumption is much more than mere fidgeting. Pharmaceutical companies and some psychiatrists have, for decades, been trying to portray restless fellow citizens who have poor concentration as ill and requiring treatment. However, never before has the myth of the hyperactive child been cultivated as passionately as it is nowadays. At least twelve different substances to be administered for the 'fidgety Philip' syndrome are currently under clinical development.[4]

What promises a turnover of billions nowadays started harmlessly: it was Frankfurt psychiatrist Heinrich Hoffmann who, in 1845, first described a nervous child in the children's book *Struwwelpeter*. Hoffmann's 'fidgety Philip' simply cannot sit still. 'He rocks his chair to and fro wriggling and squirming' – until he drags the tablecloth, crockery, cutlery, soup-bowl and all clattering to the ground. Half a century later, in the year 1902, the British medical journal *Lancet* printed an essay by a doctor who claimed to have observed children with 'inhibitory volition' and 'marked inability to concentrate and sustain attention'.[5]

However, it wasn't until decades later that ADHD's time really came. This can be dated back to an accidental laboratory finding. Leandro Panizzon, a chemist who worked for the firm Ciba, synthesised the substance methylphenidate in 1944.[6] He tried it out on himself, but did not observe any mentionable results. His wife Marguerite, known fondly as Rita, sampled the substance as well – only she felt quite an invigorating effect. From that day on, Rita occasionally took a little before her tennis match. And so the chemist Panizzon named the substance Ritalin, after his wife, Rita.

To begin with, the substance was prescribed to adults only for the treatment of excessive fatigue, depression and senile dementia; the clinical picture which would make Ritalin both famous and infamous had not yet been created.

It was not until the 1960s that new results came to light. Methylphenidate and a related substance by the name Dexedrine were having a remarkable effect on pupils with learning difficulties.

The pioneering trials were conducted by psychologist Keith Conners and psychiatrist Leon Eisenberg using Dexedrine at two schools in Baltimore, Maryland, where black children from the lower classes were educated. When the substance was distributed to the pupils, their usual high-spirited and boisterous pranks diminished. Their teachers reported an improvement in the treated children's 'classroom behaviour, attitude towards authority, and group participation' – they had found a way to make conditions at ghetto schools more bearable for themselves.[7]

These and similar results led the National Institute of Mental Health and a number of pharmaceutical companies to conduct further trials with children's pills. Soon newspapers started to report on the alleged wonder drugs, and the number of prescriptions saw a staggering rise. It remained completely unclear, however, exactly what the pills were prescribed for.

At the end of the 1960s, American doctors resolved this dilemma with a ploy to plug the lacuna, a ploy which is still in place today. The medicaments themselves could be used, so the scientists maintained, in order to diagnose the children's illness. Those who change their behaviour after taking the remedy are ill. Conversely, those children who do not respond to the substance are healthy.

This shady move paved the way for the present-day mass handout of psycho drugs to children. Until then, it would have been inconceivable to administer amphetamines and similar substances to children, just because they were behaving insubordinately at school and home. Now the situation had changed. After all, it's about curing a medical condition. The illness's existence became possible only as a result of the existence of psycho pills; the diagnosis being determined, as it is, through therapy. At the time, that is in 1970, 200,000 to 300,000 US children received behaviour-changing medications. Since then, the number – in the United States and in Germany – has risen continuously.[8]

Pharmaceutical companies called the phenomenon 'functional behavioural disorder' until the US drug-licensing agency FDA prohibited this vague designation. Promptly, the condition was renamed 'minimal brain dysfunction', and later on the notion 'hyperkinetic disorder' plagued kindergartens and primary schools. Finally in 1987, the American Psychiatry Association invented the present-day common abbreviation ADHD.

The market exploded. Nowadays, with a turnover of billions, the product name Ritalin has become the synonym for children's psycho pills. It is true that the tablets started out more expensive than the competition's. Even so, with an aggressive campaign that advertised not only the product, but the illness as well, the manufacturer secured the lead position from the very beginning. Advertisements showed classrooms with happy pupils sitting in neat rows. The teacher stands next to a boy whose face is the only blurred one on the photo. 'He is a victim of Minimal Brain Dysfunction, a diagnosable entity that generally responds well to treatment programs', the caption reads. 'And Ritalin can be an important part.'

Nowadays, the story is not dissimilar. The scene has been set in industrial nations, and a multitude of companies now competes for that lead position. All of them act as enlighteners, as far as national health is concerned – their actions aimed specifically at consolidating the ADHD phenomenon in the minds of physicians and the public.

The enterprise Medice ('Medikinet') from Iserlohn financed a specialist seminar on the subject at the German Conference of Children and Adolescent Psychiatrists March 2002 in Berlin. In unusual harmony, the competitors Medice and Novartis Pharmaceutical sponsored a supplement in the magazine *Kinder- und Jugendarzt*, which was exclusively dedicated to the topic ADHD and promoted the administering of methylphenidate.[9]

The pharmaceutical company Lilly, in turn, is the exclusive sponsor of the 'Hamburg Study Group ADD/ADHD' where a circle of dedicated medication supporters is striving to build mass nationwide awareness and has published guidelines aimed at physicians, parents and teachers. The study group, financed by this industry leader, has the teachers' best interests at heart – it wants to educate them and so is trying to get the Hamburg education authority involved in its campaign. Lilly sponsored a symposium on 'restless children and adolescents', where the chief administrative officer appeared as patron.[10]

The reason behind Lilly's financial commitment is most likely anything but selfless. Shortly, the concern wants to apply to license its own children's pill, launching an attack on the market leader Ritalin. 'Atomoxetin', the name of Lilly's substance, will improve children's 'functioning in society and family' (according to the technical journal *Ärztliche Praxis*[11]) without having as many side effects as Ritalin. In the United States, the new product is already on the market. Finally, pharmaceutical concern Janssen-Cilag has also come up with a new product: Concerta. Recently licensed in Germany, it affects children's brains for twelve hours – all day long.

While the pharmaceutical industry is sharing out the market today and tomorrow campaign by campaigns, worried parents ask themselves whether the extensive distribution of psycho pills to primary-school pupils is actually a blessing or a curse.

Paediatrician Klaus Skrodzki, practising in the Franconian town of Forchheim, is an enthusiastic proponent. 'When a child's development declines we have to intervene with medication', he says. The sprightly and multitalented man has been working for more than two decades as a general practitioner and ever-popular paediatrician. He has prescribed methylphenidate for Nina, Felix and many other children.

That Skrodzki became a German Ritalin pioneer has to do with his own son Florian, born in 1978. 'He has stood out like a sore thumb since kindergarten. His drawing was a disaster, and he was always breaking things', the father remembers. In primary school, the doctor's son could not keep up. Six weeks later the father took him out of class to see a colleague, who prescribed him methylphenidate. This was in 1985.

In spite of this intervention, his school achievements have remained modest: Florian left school without a certificate, but was later able to succeed in vocational training as a horticulturist and a fully qualified groom. Nowadays he mucks out stables and gives children riding lessons. His mother says, 'He knows how to handle horses better than people.'

His father Skrodzki continues to swear by the medical treatment of all children who are too fidgety and inattentive. 'With methylphenidate we give the child a chance to show their ability to the outside world', he says. When questioned about what was typical and unique in children with ADHD, the doctor answers: 'They can drive me round the bend here in the surgery.' Then he adds, 'But they're often much more interesting than the other children.'

For patients under six years of age Skrodzki prescribes the substance too, if he thinks it is the right thing to do – although even the manufacturers warn against this.[12] His youngest methylphenidate patient was a three-year-old. 'I feared the mother would kill the boy', was the way the doctor justified the prescription.

Paediatrician Dietrich Schultz, on the other hand, who has been practising since the mid 1980s at his Bavarian surgery, observes the extensive prescription of methylphenidate with growing unease. It is true that he has prescribed the children's pill from time to time too, because it is 'effective in certain cases'. The doctor, who is also a psychoanalyst, warns, however, that the tablets are prescribed 'much too often'. 'ADHD has been altogether artificially constructed. It is used to explain a behaviour in children which has been created by our society', Schultz argues, 'A whole generation of children is pushed into something.' Too often the pill has been administered to the youngsters without any further therapy, regrets Schultz. 'To give the medication on its own is a professional error of the doctor.' It is precisely this that critical paediatricians believe has such drastic implications for these young consumers. It can mean for them: you have a flaw in your intelligence and your emotions.

The debate that divides paediatricians echoes the opposing crusades of psychologists, therapists, teachers, mothers, fathers, grandparents and politicians. Is there a real increase in pathological behavioural abnormalities behind the en masse administering of drugs to children? Or are psycho pills used to suppress other evils that prevail in families, kindergartens and schools?

One thing is certain: disease mongers are not getting tired of portraying as many children as possible as mentally abnormal, disturbed or ill. 'Anxieties: Every seventh child needs treatment' – says a shocking headline of the German Society for Psychiatry, Psychotherapy and Mental Health. The press bulletin, which is sponsored by four pharmaceutical companies, does not mention any source for its aggressive claim.[13]

Sometimes it seems as if circumstances are enough to turn children into patients. In the opinion of psychiatrist Richard Gardner, the increasing number of divorces leads to the expansion of 'parental alienation syndrome'. That children can suffer following the separation of their parents is well known but is this suffering really a distinct illness?

The boundaries between serious disease mongering and satire are becoming blurred. In 1985, Jordan Smoller of the University of Pennsylvania wrote in a much-quoted essay that childhood 'is a syndrome which has only recently begun to receive serious attention from clinicians'. Among the most important symptoms, Smoller counts 'immaturity' and 'dwarfism'. The 'short, noisy creatures' are all too familiar to us, he says. 'The treatment of children, however, was unknown until this century, when so-called "child psychologists" and "child psychiatrists" became common.' Particularly difficult, Smoller continues, was the treatment of the so-called 'small child (or "tot")'. These children 'are known to exhibit infantile behaviour and display a startling lack of insight'.[14]

Children on drugs

The drug officer of the federal government in Germany, Marion Caspers-Merk (SPD), gets uneasy when the subject of methylphenidate comes up. 'Each year the consumption doubles', she remarks in surprised tones – and requests an inquiry into the rapid increase. Strangely enough, in 2000, the children's pill was not prescribed evenly across the federal states: it was prescribed in the city states of Bremen and Hamburg much more often than in North Rhine-Westphalia or Saxony-Anhalt.

Frequently, doctors who are not qualified to do so prescribe the psycho-pharmaceutical for children. Caspers-Merk had all methylphenidate prescriptions from 200 so-called reference chemists evaluated. Every third one had not been issued by a paediatrician or child psychiatrist, but by laboratory doctors, radiologists, ear, nose and throat specialists, gynaecologists – and in one case by a dentist. The drug officer hence suspects, 'It is not always guaranteed that a diagnosis, which leads to a methylphenidate prescription, is clear cut.'[15]

Caspers-Merk is not alone in her reservations. More and more physicians and therapists criticise the inflated prescription practice. Specialist consultants like Ulrike Lehmkuhl from Berliner Charité Hospital and Norbert Veelken from Hamburger Klinikum Nord Hospital see children time and time again who are taking methylphenidate because of a wrong diagnosis. Even if first indications of deficient attention in children are found, the use of methylphenidate is justified only for every third child.

The administering of daily medication is as indiscriminate as the alleged clinical picture is dubious. The fateful stamp – ADHD child! – is always based on the subjective impression of the doctor; the diagnostic criteria for the behaviour include attributes that can be observed in many, if not all healthy children: 'Seems often not to listen when others talk to him', 'often has difficulties organising tasks and activities', and 'often blurts out the answer.' Are these symptoms of an illness – or is this a list of behaviours, which get on (some) adults' nerves?

Doctors themselves are often at a loss and apply the already controversial diagnostic aids and guidelines haphazardly. At least one-third of all children with 'fidgety Philip' diagnosis, even by ADHD supporters' estimate, are victims of a fashionable diagnosis.[16] The arbitrary way in which children are labelled ill is also shown by cross-country comparisons. According to studies, 5.8 per cent of Brazil's children suffer from ADHD; 7.1 per cent of all children in Finland; and in the United Arab Emirates 14.9 per cent of children are allegedly unruly, attention deficient children – how such differences come about, nobody knows.[17]

In the USA, half of all the children who take methylphenidate do not have ADHD at all, even according to the diagnostic auxiliary criteria of the ADHD supporters, i.e. their standardised evaluation forms. The leading nation in attention deficient children is responsible for 80 per cent of the global methylphenidate consumption. In the United States, ADHD is as much a part of daily life as Burger King and McDonald's: around 5 million children are described as ADHD disturbed. American schools receive an annual subsidy of 400 dollars for each acknowledged patient – as compensation for the trouble with particularly rowdy pupils. In 1999 a court ruled that parents had to administer the medication to their seven-year-old son. Celltech enterprise, producer of a methylphenidate preparation, advertised its product with the promising message: 'One capsule treats ADHD for the whole school-day.'

The National Institute of Mental Health is at present financing a clinical trial in kindergartens with more than 300 children who are only just out of nappies. The test children whose ages range between three and five years are to take methylphenidate under scientific supervision for three long years.[18]

However, whether or not methylphenidate will help the children to continue to learn better in the long term is controversial, particularly since there are barely any long-term studies available. According to an inquiry from the United States, in the long run, the tablet treatment leads neither to better school achievements, nor to more manageable social behaviour.[19]

Meanwhile, physicians, therapists and parents in the United States, in Germany, and other countries around the world go on happily debating the existence and the causes of ADHD. Typical of both the complexity and range of issues are the speculations that could be heard in a crowded hall in Hamburger Klinikum Nord Hospital during a discussion evening in April 2002. A mother blamed it on contractions-suppressing drugs; a female psychologist argued there were simply no more stable boundaries in society; and the presenter, a doctor, brought up the issue of the increasing number of single mothers.

The old suspicions of chemist Hertha Hafer from Mainz, Germany, were also resurrected. In the mid 1970s, she claimed to have determined a common ingredient in foods (and by the way in the human body too) as the cause for inattentiveness: phosphates. As a test person, Hafer selected her son Herfried. The mother fed the youngster for a week with normal, phosphate-containing sausage, then another week with special sausage lacking in phosphate, and so on.

The result of the private test: when Herfried ate the phosphate-free sausage, his abnormalities, so she claimed, disappeared. Thousands believed in the phosphate theory. At the slaughterhouse in Hamburg worried parents gathered from 6 a.m. They wanted to buy completely fresh meat – believing that it would contain less phosphate. That this 'phosphate diet' could never be proven scientifically has not affected its popularity: Hafer's book on the subject is in its sixth edition.[20]

The latest ADHD craze features the bacterial mush 'Afa-algae'. The Federal Institute for Consumer Health Protection in Germany has warned strongly against this remedy. There is 'no scientific proof' for its claimed healing power. Furthermore, the bacteria might contain toxins, which is why 'children should categorically not consume any Afa-algae products'.

Even though no doctor is able to recognise an ADHD affected person based on his or her brain structure, one expert opinion that has become popular in recent years describes the condition as a biological disorder.[21] However, even with imaging procedures it is not possible to differentiate diagnostically between the brains of hyperactive and normal children.

ADHD – a legacy from the Stone Age?

Scientists claim to have found striking evidence concerning ADHD's origins – evidence which has become warped into crude theories by some pharmaceutical companies. The special brochure 'Inattentive and hyperactive' of *Kinderärztliche Praxis* magazine (financially supported by Novartis) speculates that hyperactivity is a legacy from the Stone Age: 'The ADHD symptomatology can be regarded as having been an advantageous genetic predisposition in previous times; however, it becomes a disadvantage in today's modern society and endangers children's development and adaptation.'[22]

Such speculations find sympathetic listeners in parents of inattentive children – because they can acquit themselves of the charge of having failed with their upbringing. A collective sigh of relief was heard for example at the discussion evening in Hamburg, when a doctor claimed, 'It is rubbish to say that ADHD develops through upbringing.'

After having asked themselves for years what they've done wrong, mothers and fathers find consolation in the spreading belief that ADHD is as innate a phenomenon as being born with earlobes attached to the head. Franconian school teacher Irene Braun, whose son – now fully grown – has been taking Ritalin for years, also believes in the power of genes. She says, 'My son was already showing anomalous signs prior to his birth, he used to kick me inside the womb.' Little Felix's mother is also certain that her son suffers from an innate metabolic disorder, 'He is lacking a messenger agent in the brain.'

Physicians and biologists do agree, though, that ADHD cannot be traced back to the malfunctioning of a single gene. It is rather the case that a still unknown multitude of genes influences a child's temperament and ability to concentrate.

This is precisely why the new fashionable view that ADHD is innate does not release parents from their duty: only the child's upbringing, family and environment decide whether and to what degree a genetic disposition to being a fidgety Philip actually develops into a trait. Child psychiatrists like Benno Schimmelmann from the University Hospital Eppendorf in Hamburg hence talk at best about a 'genetic vulnerability'.

However, many of the affected parents do not want to hear anything about such complicated, yet important subtleties. Accordingly, the pharmaceutical industry is making every effort to portray ADHD as a purely biological disorder, which can be treated conveniently with a pill. The Medikinet producer, for instance, claims impertinently in advertisements: Methylphenidate 'stimulates neurotransmitter metabolism'.

Until quite recently, very little was known about what methylphenidate actually does in the developing brains of children. Although the substance has been administered to restless patients for fifty years, it was not until the summer of 2001 that psychiatrist Nora Volkow from Brookhaven National Laboratory in New York found indications as to what methylphenidate triggers in the brain: The substance blocks certain transport proteins, thus increasing the concentration of the messenger agent dopamine in the synapses – hence, it has an effect comparable to the drug cocaine.[23]

Methylphenidate leaves traces in the brain

It is true that methylphenidate seems to be non-addictive if taken in tablet form. Indeed, it takes effect much more slowly than cocaine and does not create the same 'kick'. However, the substance, being an amphetamine, does fall under the regulations of the narcotic law. As mentioned before, in Germany it has to be prescribed according to the same restrictive guidelines as morphine, for example, with three copies of the prescription and the regulation that these must be kept on record for ten years.

Among the side effects that can be expected when taking Ritalin, the psychomotor states of excitement, anxiety, insomnia and paranoia appear on the German Federation of Pharmaceutical Industries' 'Red List'. After abrupt discontinuation of long-term treatment, patients can be plagued by withdrawal symptoms. In addition, the medicine spoils many children's appetite: seven-year-old Jasmine from the Schleswig-Holstein town of Norderstedt was to experience just how severe the side effects can be. 'She got nervous twitches in her hands, bit her lips till they became bloody, and in the evenings she doubled up with stomach aches in her bed', says the father. After three months, he released his daughter from Ritalin and is now desperately looking for an alternative therapy. Finally, it is feared that the daily dose of methylphenidate may disturb the growth of children. According to a study, long-term consumers remain 1.5 centimetres shorter than other children over a two-year period.[24]

The fear of possible long-term consequences makes many doctors, and parents as well, shrink from administering the psycho drug. The medicaments alter the structural conditions in which a child's brain develops. One thing is uncontroversial: that methylphenidate leaves lasting traces in the brain. Thus, the substance influences which genes in the nerve cells are switched on and off. A group of researchers conducting animal experiments under the supervision of neuroscientist Gerald Hüther from Göttingen found modifications in the brains of rodents. The researchers gave young rats methylphenidate, let them grow up and examined their brains: in a small region of the brain, the number of dopamine transporters was half what it should have been.[25]

This might lead, according to Hüther, to a dopamine deficiency – and thereby trigger Parkinson's in the long run. If we give methylphenidate to children, warns the scientist in an often quoted, controversial article, then we run the 'risk of enhancing the very conditions for the development' of the dreaded tremor paralysis.[26] Characteristic of the dispute about methylphenidate is Aribert Rothenberger, Hüther's colleague of all people, who examined the rat brains together with him, yet distanced himself from the fear-arousing interpretation. Hüther's warnings drew their power of conviction from a 'mixture of speculations and half-truths', wrote the director of the Child and Adolescent Psychiatric Clinic Göttingen in an open letter to parents, who had become completely insecure.

American political scientist Francis Fukuyama opposes the increasing medicalisation of childhood problems more adamantly than others. In the USA not only methylphenidate, but also medicaments against anxieties and psychoses, mood stabilisers and antidepressants are nowadays prescribed to twice as many children and adolescents as they were only a decade previously. The drug agency FDA licensed the so-called happiness pill Prozac for young people between 7 and 17 years of age who are depressive and difficult.[27] Fukuyama condemns this flood of pills and advocates more courage in bringing up children. 'It is hard to make a brief in favour of pain and suffering', he admits. Nevertheless, children had to learn, he adds, how to cope without psycho pills, even at times of emotional distress. It is only through the experience of the depths of human suffering that opposite '"good" emotions' like sympathy, compassion, courage and solidarity may emerge. Fukuyama criticises any pharmaceutical therapy for the soul. Modern society was running the risk of robbing itself of development if it kept trying, by means of psycho-pharmaceuticals, to create a steady, always functioning human being. The whole 'range of more nuanced feelings of discontent and discomfort may also be the source of creativity, wonder and innovation'.

In the eyes of Fukuyama, methylphenidate is a mere 'technology of social control'. The medicine eases 'the burden of parents and teachers while relieving those diagnosed with ADHD of responsibility for their own condition'. It was once believed that 'character was something that had to be shaped through self-discipline, struggle and a willing-ness to commit chromatrous and comply incommiant, antorpmion nomi plains, 'now we have a medical shortcut to get the same result'.[28]

Children could indeed get other kinds of help, for example through simple lifestyle changes. The story of a young Englishman who went to school at the end of the nineteenth century and who most probably would have been classified as hyperactive based on present-day criteria might provide an example. To get rid of his superfluous energy, the restless soul arranged with his teachers to be allowed to run around the school building after each lesson. Thereby, school life became indeed more bearable – for both pupil and teachers. In his later life, however, the Englishman refrained from further sporting activities. His name – Winston Churchill.[29]

7 The femininity syndrome

On 27 July 1872, gynaecology came to a bloody turning point. Alfred Hegar, professor of obstetrics and gynaecology in Freiburg, removed the intact ovaries of a 27-year-old woman from Kenzingen, because she had complained about abdominal pain during her menstruation. The woman 'herself demanded the operation after having been treated for two years without success with all kinds of localised remedies as well as other cures that affect the whole body'.[1] A few days after the incision, the patient was dead; she died of a peritoneum inflammation.

The castration with deadly consequences marks the beginning of an aggressive gynaecology. Previously, gynaecologists had practised a gentler medicine, but based on surgical progress during the nineteenth century, they began to perform major operations. Ovariectomy, that is the removal of one or both ovaries, was, in the beginning, particularly popular. Cutting out the womb (hysterectomy) soon became a procedure that also enriched the repertoire of gynaecologists.

These amputations were meant to treat physical complaints, but often mental problems were also implicated. In the years between 1850 and 1900, a whole school of gynaecologists and psychiatrists supported the opinion that 'pathological states and processes in the female genitals can cause madness', as German gynaecologist Louis Mayer put it.[2] The best way to cure this pudenda-conditioned madness was a radical operation.

Since these obscure beginnings, gynaecology has become an even wider field. Nowadays, women's natural transition phases are all considered medical problems: puberty, pregnancy, childbirth, the days before her monthly period, menstruation itself and last but not least menopause. 'The crucial point in this context is not the fact that female patients can get medicine for the treatment of diseases and relief of problems', states psychologist Petra Kolip, but that the boundaries between healthy and sick have shifted so that bodily processes, which were previously 'normal' per definition, are now regarded as pathological, which means that the intervention realm of medicine is expanding – needless to say, not always in the patients' best interest.[3]

Even childlessness is considered a disease; at any rate, the national health services pay for the first advances into the labyrinth of reproduction medicine. Techniques that are ever more ingenious have been developed in recent years to fulfil couples' dreams of having a child of their own. On average every fifty minutes, somewhere in Germany an artificially procreated baby is born.

One of the earliest occurrences of the term 'medicalisation' was in the context of gynaecology, in an article published in 1970 in the *New England Journal of Medicine*. It deals with the topic of how sexually active female teenagers are treated by doctors: they inspect body, genitals and teeth; they examine blood and urine values. This is followed by a house call by a nurse. Already then, it said, this represented 'a "medicalisation" of sex that is probably self-defeating'.[4]

Sentenced for life – at the gynaecologist

By now, it seems a matter of course that girls go to the doctor as soon as their periods start – just to check if 'everything is in order'. These early ties with medicine did not come about out of the blue: in 1978 a so-called 'study group for child and teenage gynaecology' was founded to attract a certain clientele. In the past, pharmaceutical companies advised gynaecologists through brochures about implementing special surgery hours for teenagers – in order to tie tomorrow's women as early as possible to the practice. Nowadays, companies are approaching teenage girls directly, for example through free magazines that are displayed at gynaecological surgeries. 'When arranging an appointment, please ask for the teen consultation scheme', the magazine *Women's Health* advises; it is published, according to the imprint, with 'exclusive support from the Grünenthal Co. Ltd'. The editorial says, 'Gynaecologists become companions through all stages of life and often they develop a life-long relationship with their patients – from their youth through to old age.'[5]

The first consultation in the stirrups is discussed in feminist circles as an initiation rite in the western world. Sociologist Eva Schindele sees girls' first gynaecologist appointment as 'an introduction into a culture where their femininity is defined and examined by men'.[6]

In fact, most of the time it is indeed male doctors who determine which of women's bodily processes and conditions are to be described as illnesses. As early as the end of the 1960s an American doctor named Wright pleaded, as a preventive measure, to remove the uterus of older women: 'The uterus becomes a useless, bleeding, trouble-making, possibly cancer-producing organ, which therefore should be removed.'[7]

Removal of the uterus is nowadays the most common incision that is performed on women during the second half of their life. 'It seems as if the loss of the uterus were almost part of menopause, as if the uterus were to become from a certain moment in a woman's life onwards a useless organ', reflects health scientist Klaus Müller.[8]

In Germany around 160,000 uteruses are removed each year – though according to experts at least 60,000 of these operations are superfluous. Only 10 to 15 per cent of all cases deal with the preven-tion or elimination of serious or life-threatening diseases like cancer. Frequent indications include heavy or irregular menstruation as well as aches and cramps in the lower abdomen. However, these symptoms may also occur if diagnosis does not lead to any pathological results, as a UK study shows. Women who had undergone a hysterectomy because of irregular periods were examined. It turned out, however, that 40 per cent of the amputated organs were completely healthy.[9]

Benign tumours in the uterus wall emerge during the fourth decade of life in approximately every fifth woman. The emergence of such myomas is the most frequent cause for surgical intervention. The growth of these tumours is encouraged by the sexual hormone oestrogen. Because the body's own production of oestrogen decreases during menopause, the growth of myomas comes to a halt, and some-times they even disappear. This beneficent bodily process stops func-tioning when menopause is suspended by hormone replacement therapy. Through constant oestrogen supply the myomas are able to grow further so that 'from a certain size and coverage onwards surgical removal of the uterus becomes inevitable because of pain and harm to neighbouring organs', Müller says. The medicalisation of menopause thereby leads to a real disease as a consequence.

The number of hysterectomies is directly determined by the needs of physicians. For further medical education and specialisation, gynaecol-ogists in Germany previously had to have performed approximately thirty hysterectomies. Later on, the education module no longer included these compulsory operations – and promptly fewer organs were cut out. In France, for example, hysterectomies are much rarer than in Germany.[10] The differences have a cultural background.

French clinicians have a more holistic treatment approach and aspire to preserve the whole of the body, the so-called *terrain*.

It is therefore a fact that physicians' habits and preferences are a more crucial factor than medical necessities in deciding whether a woman's womb is to go or not.

A new periodic system

'Woman's anguish has seized my body, so let the gods free me from this evil' – this is what a Babylonian woman carved into a clay tablet around 3,000 BC.[11] Woman's longing for the end of all periods is now becoming an impending reality. Not gods, but physicians have decided to put an end to menstruation. They do not see a medical reason for this natural process any longer. 'It is a needless loss of blood', writes Brazilian reproductive biologist Elsimar Coutinho.[12] Moreover, the regular bleeding was even detrimental to woman's health. 'Many women have challenging and difficult lives [and can't be bothered with menstruation]', declares medical doctor David Grimes from the University of Northern California.[13] There was therefore good reason for them to avoid their period if they liked.

The new cycle is easy. If women take daily hormone dosages in the form of common contraceptives, without interruption, they can suppress menstruation for months and even years. However, the pill packages are designed to last for twenty-one days; after that, one stops taking the pills or takes only pills which do not contain the active ingredient. Then the hormone level drops rapidly, and the woman starts to have bleedings. These withdrawal bleedings have little to do with the original menstruation and in many women – as a side effect of the pill – they fail to appear.

Elsimar Coutinho and his fellows want to turn this exception into the rule. Women will take the pill no longer for birth control, but so they may enjoy a more convenient and allegedly healthier life without periods. They portray menstruation as women's worst scourge. Moreover, the doubtlessly existing aches and feelings of utter discomfort during menstruation ('dysmenorrhoea') are topped off by the allegedly arduous episodes before the period, the 'premenstrual syndrome'.

The first anti-period products are already available. Hormone packages that are put under the skin and depot injections suppress bleedings for many weeks. The preparation 'Seasonale', which the American firm Barr Laboratories wants to launch, functions in a similar way. The medicine contains the active ingredient of the good old pill, but it would grant women a cycle of ninety-one days: eighty-four days of hormone intake, then seven sugar pills – the female consumers would bleed only four times a year. Pharmaceutical researchers find this frequency conducive to promoting life quality and career chances of women.[14]

'Once patients and physicians understand the benefits, this is going to be the way to take the pill', says gynaecologist Patricia Sulak of the Department of Obstetrics and Gynaecology at Texas A&M University. Her career goal is 'to eliminate monthly periods'.[15]

For their attack on monthly periods, researchers declare present-day woman as an ailing product of evolution. It is unnatural that women in industrial countries have 450 menstruations throughout their lifespan. Prehistoric women had, it is said, only 160 monthly periods. However, the comparison is poor. On the one hand, the latter had a much shorter life expectancy; on the other hand, they were pregnant more often.

An illness named pregnancy

In Germany, 'being expectant' brings medicine on to the scene to an increasing degree. Thus, the number of medical examinations for pregnant women has increased since the mid 1980s by 500 per cent, as sociologist Eva Schindele calculated.[16] Moreover, to have a 'risk pregnancy' is from the viewpoint of statistics almost regarded as normal – more than half of the expectant mothers are now classified in this way.

Pregnant women, though, have not become less healthy in recent years at all. The boom of risks goes back to the physicians' zeal: they apply ever-higher standards to the natural event of pregnancy. During a completely normal pregnancy development, a woman has to present herself ten times to the doctor. Every couple of weeks, weight is recorded, blood pressure measured, urine examined, blood analysed. The womb, the embryo's heartbeat and the position of the unborn child are all subjected to medical supervision. Whosoever differs from standard values that are, after all, arbitrarily determined, gets a small cross sign under the heading of 'risk pregnancy' in her pregnancy record booklet.

Nowadays, these booklets contain a list of fifty-two different risk categories. First-time mothers under 18 and over 35 years are regarded as being at risk from the outset. The same applies to women whose weight is 20 per cent above the weight defined as normal. Events like previous births by Caesarean section, multiple children at one birth and birth of a disabled child incite the special care of medicine. And last but not least, gynaecologists themselves become a risk-increasing factor. With the density of practices the number of risk pregnancies actually rises as well, as was shown by an investigation in the Saarland. The profusion of risk factors undermines pregnant women's sense of security. It could be that – in the sense of a self-fulfilling prophecy – It is precisely this that leads, in some cases, to actual complications. At any rate, more calmness and composure do not do any harm before childbirth. In Scandinavia and the Netherlands, the proportion of risk pregnancies is only around 20 per cent, probably because midwives play a bigger role in preventive healthcare there than elsewhere. In the Netherlands, anaesthesia, the carefully performed perineal cut and other procedures are the exception during normal births even in hospitals. The rate of Caesarean sections is only 10 per cent – and infant mortality is as low as in Germany.

Without labour into the world

> Victoria Beckham, 27, knows exactly when her second child will be born: on the first of September. According to the *Mirror* 'Posh Spice' has chosen this date for her planned Caesarean section at a private London clinic, because it fits perfectly in between two of David Beckham's football matches.
> (*Süddeutsche Zeitung*, 19 August 2002)

> Romeo Beckham is here. The second son of Spice Girl Victoria and football star David Beckham saw the light of day yesterday.
> (*Süddeutsche Zeitung*, 2 September 2002)

Twenty minutes anaesthesia, a small cut through the abdominal wall – and already the infant is lying in his mother's arms. The previously much feared Caesarean has become trendy: 43.2 per cent of German women would opt for this.[17] The rate of Caesareans is increasing tremendously: from 6 per cent at the beginning of the 1980s to 20 per cent most recently, and at German university clinics even up to 28 per cent.

It is true that most of the sections are still performed because doctors regard the well-being of the child or mother to be at risk. However, approximately 6 to 8 per cent of women do choose to have an operation. 'There are couples who come to consult me, and they're asking right away for information about Caesarean section', says Hans-Jürgen Kitschke, director of the women's clinic in Offenbach.[18]

The first Caesarean section, which mother and child survived, is said to have been carried out in the year 1500 in the Swiss town of

Siegershausen by a man named Jakob Nufer. The man was a master in the use of sharp knifes – after all, his profession was castrating pigs (emasculated pigs accumulate fat faster). His wife had spent several days in labour and thirteen midwives as well as several doctors had reached the end of their wits. It was then that castrator Nufer took action. A handed down document describes the act: 'Then the man locked the door, called upon god almighty for help and support, put his wife on the table and cut her belly open (as it is done to pigs)'.

According to the written record, the desperate action had a happy ending. 'The very first cut into the belly was so fortunate and well-performed that the infant was soon extracted unharmed and in one piece.' The wound of the mother was stitched, as one does when 'mending old shoes'. The woman recovered.[19]

After this single anecdotal event, the section remained for centuries a horror story. In nineteenth-century Europe, only 14 per cent of women survived the belly cutting. Gynaecologist Edoardo Porro from Milan changed this situation by introducing a new method in 1876. He cut the child out together with the uterus and so was able to stop the bleeding. As a result, at least half of the women survived the section.

Until a couple of years ago, the path 'inter faeces et urinam' (between excrement and urine) was regarded the ideal way into life. In the 1970s, only three to five out of a hundred children in industrial nations were born by Caesarean section. And hospitals where doctors took to the scalpel particularly often gained a bad reputation: apparently, the art of obstetrics was not being mastered in their delivery rooms. Delivery by incision was regarded as dangerous, and a mother who had to deliver her baby by section was pitied – she would 'miss' the birth of her 'cut-out-offspring' in full anaesthesia. Moreover, she would have to lie in a hospital bed with an aching scar for up to two weeks.

Among Brazil's upper class it is nowadays considered unsophisticated to give birth through the vagina – in Rio 85 out of 100 women have a Caesarean and preserve the 'vagina of a teenager'. In the Mexican city of Monterey, expectant mothers get birth documents for their children including date of birth in advance. 'In countries of the former Soviet Union, something like 96 per cent of births are natural. It's cultural. The people are used to tolerate pain. Here they are not.'[20] In the United States, every third pregnant woman with private health insurance adheres to the slogan 'Preserve your love channel – take a Caesarean.' And in Thailand, many women decide to have their baby delivered by section so the child can be born on the day predicted by a fortune-teller.

In the *British Medical Journal* experts state that in recent years, birth has moved away from being a normal physiological process and towards becoming a 'medical event under the supervision of a gynaecologist'.[21] (Interestingly, psychiatrists are trying to make a profit from the technicalisation of birth. Under the heading, 'The birth event as trauma' the German Society for Psychiatry, Psychotherapy and Neurology claims that after a Caesarean section, many mothers were afflicted by 'severe and long lasting depressions'. Moreover, 'long-term breastfeeding problems and crying babies can be the result'.)

A survey among medically trained midwives showed that 31 per cent would deliver by Caesarean even if they had a problem-free pregnancy with a single baby. 'Birth per section has today become a serious "treatment alternative" to vaginal birth', comments Peter Husslein from the University Women's Clinic in Vienna. 'Hence, it has to be the goal of modern obstetrics to enable every woman, as far as possible, to have her desired birth.'[22]

There is strong competition among the delivery rooms, because fewer and fewer babies are being born. This is also the reason doctors are accommodating pregnant women beyond medical necessity. 'Anyone who offers women the most comfortable birth', says gynaecologist Kitschke from Offenbach, 'often receives an additional payment, and health insurance pays double for Caesarean-section births'. A section costs on average 1,500 Euros more than a normal birth.

The World Health Organisation considers a section rate of 15 per cent acceptable based on medical criteria (as a reminder, for comparison, the rate in Germany is 20 per cent). A surplus of medicine beyond this does not lead to better health at all. In the Netherlands and in Sweden the rate is 10 to 12 per cent, without jeopardising the health of mothers and children.

Conversely, the Caesarean-to-order holds bigger risks than normal birth. Around 20 per cent of mothers electing for a section develop a fever because their wound gets inflamed. In addition, 2 per cent of babies, who take the seemingly easy way out, come into contact with the scalpel and are born with a scratch.[23] In spite of all the progress in surgical and anaesthetic techniques, twice as many women still die during Caesareans than during normal birth. Statistically, one out of 17,000 mothers dies after a section; one out of 47,000 after a vaginal birth.[24] Also, delivery per section is a heavier burden on the health system. When the number of Caesareans rises in Germany by 1 per cent, there is a dramatic increase in expenditure. Birgit Seelbach-Göbel, consultant at the Women's Clinic St. Hedwig in Regensburg, says, 'The consequence can actually only be that expectant women will have to pay for elective sections.'[25]

Even so, the triumphant march of the Caesarean seems to have become unstoppable. In the spring of 2002, the German Society for Gynaecology and Obstetrics also licensed the 'accommodation section'. A relating statement says 'where medical indication for section is not applicable, but where there is no contra-indication either, the obstetrician is allowed to comply with the serious and urgent wish of the woman to have a delivery by Caesarean.'[26]

Magical elixir from mare's pee

Menopause might be a natural phase in the life of a woman, but the medical establishment never thought of it as beneficial. 'The years of the climacteric are the most troublesome in married life', declared Slovakian doctor Arnold Lorand back in the year 1910, 'not only for the wife, who is directly affected by it, but also in almost equal degree for the husband, who must show the greatest forbearance.' Lorand himself is believed to have found a cure for the troubled years of the climacteric. Extracts from sows' ovaries could 'put off old age for a score of years' or at least 'mitigate its effects when it has asserted itself with all its terrors'.

A little later, in the 1940s, pharmaceutical companies extracted the much sought-after oestrogen in large quantities, not from pigs, but from pregnant mares' urine (a well-known product name is derived from pregnant mares' urine: Premarine). In 1960 the *New England Journal of Medicine* recommended hormones for 'everyone with evidence of an oestrogen lack' – which meant almost every woman over 50.

But it was not until the mid 1960s with the publication of the bestseller *Feminine Forever* in the United States that animal sex hormones were turned into mass drugs.[27] In his book, the young New Yorker gynaecologist Robert Wilson described the stuff made from mare's pee as magical medicine, promising eternal youth. 'For the first time in history women may share the promise of tomorrow as biological equals of men . . . thanks to hormone therapy, they may look forward to prolonged well-being and extended youth.'

Wilson fulfilled his mission also towards the medical profession. 'At age 50, there are no ova, no follicles, no theca, no oestrogen – truly a galloping catastrophe', he wrote in the *Journal of the American Geriatric Society* in 1972. But oestrogen could save these women: 'Breasts and genital organs will not shrivel. Such women will be much more pleasant to live with and will not become dull and unattractive.'28

What nobody knew back then was that the pharmaceutical firm Wyeth Ayerst had paid Wilson's expenses for his work on the book. Later on, it also sponsored his 'Wilson Research Foundation', which had its offices in Manhattan's Park Avenue. Moreover, it paid Robert Wilson to give women's groups talks about his hormone primer.

It was not until 2002 that Wilson's son Ronald made these involvements public. Wyeth, as the pharmaceutical firm is now called, had by then become the biggest hormone manufacturer in the world. Dr Barbara Wanner from Zurich comments: 'It is evident that the definition of menopause as a disease emerged exactly at the same time synthetic hormones became available to treat this newly defined disease.'29

Millions of women fell for the propaganda. Oestrogen was portrayed as vital stuff – the fact that many women survive forty more years of life without it was not mentioned. In 1981, even the WHO gave in to the new definition of menopause – and described it as an oestrogen deficiency disease. That many women, however, live healthily until old age, and on average much longer than men do, is a fact that did not receive any further discussion.

Nowadays, taking hormones is, for older women in the western world, part of everyday life. Around 4.6 million women over 45 in Germany alone take the preparations. They seem to have either forgotten or never to have heard about the cancer suspicion, which circulated for the first time in the mid 1970s. Two extensive studies indicated at the time that oestrogen increased the risk of developing cancer of the uterus. However, this could not stop the career of the hormones. Physicians and producers swiftly presented a new combination preparation made from oestrogen and the corpus luteum hormone progesterone, which is supposedly harmless and non-carcinogenic. However, in the mid 1990s, these combination drugs themselves gained a bad reputation. It became ever more evident that this hormone mix increases the risk of breast cancer.

But on this occasion too, pharmaceutical firms and gynaecologists succeeded, once again, in dispelling any worries. At the end of 2000, the German Society for Gynaecology and Obstetrics as well as six further specialist societies claimed:

> Mortality rate of postmenopausal women is reduced by about 50 per cent through hormone replacements, which can be attributed primarily to the advantageous effect that oestrogen

preparations have on the heart and cardiovascular system. Even the mortality rate related to carcinomas can be reduced by around 30 per cent if hormone replacements are taken.[30]

Millions of women trusted doctors and innocently kept taking their prescribed hormones.

Yet the artificially supplied preparations intervene in a natural transformation process of the body. Already four years before the actual menopause, the concentration of the various hormones in the body starts to fluctuate. During the actual years of the climacteric – on average when women are around 50 years old – the body reduces its production of oestrogen as well as of gestagen, the pregnancy hormone. Oestrogen is the most important female hormone; it affects the genital organs, directs the monthly cycle and affects bone structure. Some women experience this phase as uncomfortable: they experience night sweats and hot flushes, circulatory problems, insomnia, vaginal dryness and nervousness.

Hot flushes unknown in Japan

What doctors in the western world call 'menopause-syndrome' is almost unknown in Japan. When Margaret Lock from McGill University in Montreal investigated the phenomenon in Japan, her questions were met with lack of understanding. Among 1,225 questioned women around 50 years of age, only 15 per cent reported night sweats and hot flushes. Japanese gynaecologists declare the climacteric and its troubles coolly as a problem of the west. Only a few indolent women from Japan's upper class have recently started to make their lives miserable with this *idée fixe* – a fashionable disease.[31]

In Germany, on the other hand, anyone who resists hormone replacement therapy is regarded as unreasonable. Administering oestrogen or a combination of oestrogen and gestagen has become part of standard medicine; it costs German health insurance 500 million Euros a year. There seems to be at least one proven benefit of short-term hormone intake. Many women already feel better because their complaints are taken seriously and they can walk away with a pill to be cured.

In the mid 1980s, menopausal woman was depicted as sickly, wizened and depressive. Physicians and pharmaceutical companies, however, could not content themselves with prescribing hormones only for those women who felt uncomfortable. Since the 1980s, they have been painting a new picture of the climacteric. Menopause is depicted less as a troublesome phase, but as a risk for a whole range of diseases. This shift is clearly visible in the advertising approach of the industry. Now, 'menopausal woman' appears as a healthy and spruce creature, whose enviable state is however threatened! To stay healthy, so the enticing call goes, older women should take hormones – preferably for the rest of their lives. 'This new message has already hit its target', says Dr Barbara Wanner, 'there are already healthy women coming to our surgery enquiring about risks.'[32]

In recent years, doctors have celebrated the hormone preparations as true miracle cures. In the autumn of 1991 for example, epidemiologists from Harvard Medical School in Boston reported a legendary protective effect of oestrogen. Their ten-year trial which included 48,470 nurses seemed to show that taking oestrogen reduced the risk of suffering a cardiac infarct by almost a half. Head of the study, Meir Stampfer, was rapturous: 'That is why healthy postmenopausal women should also take oestrogen.'

At the same time, a group of researchers at the University Women's Clinic in Ulm attempted to dispel the often-evoked risk of increased development of breast cancer and tumours in the mucous membrane of the uterus after long-term oestrogen intake. The group around Christian Lauritzen announced that precisely this risk could be avoided by taking the usual prescription of combined oestrogen-gestagen preparations. The clinicians had observed 1,402 women over a period of twenty-one years. Moreover, if both female sex hormones were taken in small dosages, the frequency of cancer was even reduced.

Full of optimism, the physicians from Ulm addressed the public. It was finally proven that the 'long-term oestrogen replacement has tremendous advantages: The whole metabolism is positively affected'. When treating women in their menopause, practising gynaecologists in their surgeries should do more often than before 'what we doctors do otherwise every day – correcting nature'.[33]

The euphoria reached new heights. Oestrogen, it was said, would help relieve age-related bone atrophy (osteoporosis), Alzheimer's and even intestinal cancer too. It was a cost-effective means to prevent chronic diseases. Those women, however, who remained sceptical, were often regarded as irresponsible – towards society too. In Switzerland, pharmaceutical firm Janssen-Cilag provided doctors with colour transparencies for their menopausal women consultations, which claimed that hormone replacement therapy reduced the risk of bone fractures by 75 per cent, the risk of developing Alzheimer's by 54 per cent and the risk of cardiovascular diseases by 44 per cent.[34]

In 1996, Professor Christian Lauritzen from Ulm, an opinion-maker who had a strong influence on his medical practitioner colleagues, put some more wood on the fire:

> The extensive prevention of oestrogen deficiency's long-term consequences (such as osteoporosis fractures, cardiac infarct and stroke), made possible through long-term administering of oestrogen, is undoubtedly one of the most important advances in preventive medicine over the last decade.[35]

Physician Herbert Kuhl from Frankfurt even went so far as to urge the licensing authorities indirectly to moderate the warnings on the user information leaflets in the drug packaging. These warnings would only lead women to refuse the hormones or discontinue their use prematurely. In 1994, Kuhl complained in the journal *Deutsches Ärzteblatt*: 'These restrictions have disadvantageous effects on the prevention of common diseases such as osteoporosis, arteriosclerosis and cardiac infarct.'[36]

Nevertheless, the references to the healing power of hormones were not at all based on hard scientific evidence. Some of the favourable results go back to the so-called 'healthy user' effect: women who are on long-term hormones, are often more health aware, have fewer risk factors and are from the start in a better state of health than others.

Myth of beneficent hormones pops

In the United States, the Wyeth firm wanted, in 1990, to have its hormone products officially acknowledged as a drug that helps prevent heart diseases. An advisory committee of the drug licensing authority FDA had already agreed to the request, but in-house sceptics overruled the supporters in the end. They demanded to see precise data and advised the applicant to carry out a clinical trial.

Wyeth started a study that would not – or that was not supposed to – leave any room for doubt. The women were divided into two groups – none of them knew whether she was taking a hormone or a placebo; 2,763 women with an existing heart condition and an average age of 67 participated in the experiment. Most of the clinicians and pharmaceutical researchers were confident of victory: the carefully planned study ('heart and oestrogen/progestin replacement study', in short 'Hers') would confirm the beneficent effect of hormones on the heart.

But things were to take a different turn. After the first year of the study, in 1998, a disadvantageous effect on the infarct rate began to emerge. The women treated with hormones clearly suffered more often from complications than those who had taken the placebo drug. The hope, that the hormones would start to protect the heart after long-term application, was lost. A subsequent study (Hers-2) was also called off. The outcome after almost seven years is sobering: the oestrogen preparations do not benefit heart health at all.[37]

In July 2002, a report followed that filled millions of women in America and Europe with disbelief and horror. In the United States, another study analysing the effect of hormones on 16,000 women was cut short – to protect the health of the test persons. For an interim evaluation had shown that the hormone preparations had done *damage* rather than given benefit.[38]

This study, initially scheduled to continue until 2005 (Women's Health Initiative: WHI), was supposed to prove, in turn, the benefit of hormones and to base the long-term administering of oestrogen preparations finally on scientifically solid foundations. Instead, the clinicians discovered dangerous side effects: when 10,000 women take a combination preparation (oestrogen and gestagen) for a year, there will be among them eight more cases of breast cancer than in a comparative group of women who do not take hormones. Of 10,000, seven more will suffer a cardiac infarct, eight more will have a stroke and eight more will have a blood clot. However, advantages were also noted. Six fewer cases of intestinal cancer and five fewer cases of broken hip joints can be expected.

Whether the instances of diseases were initially related to oestrogen is a question which the study cannot answer. Oestrogen does seem to slow down the age-related bone atrophy, osteoporosis. That this actually prevents bone fractures is still unproven. After weighing advantages and disadvantages, American doctors decided to call off the study. They advised women: 'Do not use oestrogen-gestagen combinations to prevent chronic diseases.'

Hormone specialist Martina Dören from Berliner University Clinic Benjamin Franklin went even further: the concept of hormone replacement therapy was, after the study, 'shaken, if not finished'.

Some of her medical colleagues, though, had a different view. The competent committee of the Association of Gynaecologists hastily compiled a two-page text addressing the 'dear patient' and signed it 'your gynaecologist's practice'. The letter was sent to the 11,000 members – to be precise via fax from pharmaceutical companies Jenapharm and Schering, which sell hormone preparations with a turnover of several millions.[39]

The committee of gynaecologists embellished the results as if they had been written by the marketing department of the pharmaceutical companies. The WHI study's clearly proven *increase* in cardiac infarct and stroke is dismissed as 'no reduction in cardiovascular diseases'. And as far as breast cancer risk is concerned, the authors argue disgracefully that the accelerated growth of tumours was in fact a blessing. They are trying to make women in the waiting room believe:

> The recovery chances for tumours that develop under oestrogen therapy are clearly better. Since hormone-treated women have regular gynaecological examinations, these tumours may be discovered earlier so that they can be removed in most of the cases without jeopardizing the breast.

Perfidiously, disease mongers want to earn twice. They fight menopause with hormones, and later, they cut out the tumours that develop as a consequence.

The US study with 16,000 women could not even confirm the repeatedly claimed positive influence of oestrogen-gestagen preparations on general well-being. In March 2003, the authors revealed to the public a disillusioning result. The hormone taking had no measurable influence on the general state of health, nor on vitality, mental condition, depressive episodes or sexual satisfaction.[40]

The medicalisation of the menopause is an example par excellence of the way certain physicians' groups and pharmaceutical firms are manipulating the evidence in medical issues. Nowadays menopausal woman is regarded as a deficient being. Lower Saxony's subdivision of the Association of Gynaecologists claims defiantly, 'Menopause is a disease.'[41] Physicians and pharmaceutical companies have launched half-truths, legends and advice that led millions of healthy women to take oestrogen and gestagen. Scientific proof for the benefit of hormone preparations is still not available.

Doctors and chemists who publish the independent *arznei-telegramm* are demanding something that should be in fact a matter of course: that 'on principle only those medicaments which have proven efficiency and safety according to sufficiently extensive, controlled and randomised long-term studies should be used'.[42]

Women's health seems to have vanished, washed away by unrelenting tides of disease – as one ebbs so the next advances. One is almost inclined to believe that to be of the female sex has become a disease in itself. The years of menstruation are followed by menopause, which is followed in turn by years of hormone deficiency. Only childhood and earliest youth are regarded as symptom-free stages.

8   Old men, new afflictions

A new disease is threatening the stronger sex – the male menopause. Schuster Public Relations & Media Consulting Firm identified the danger: 'Of men in their "prime" two-thirds have health complaints', it warned the German public in October 2002. 'When they "reach middle age", mood swings, sleeping disorders and other "climacteric troubles" cause men trouble too. That a testosterone deficiency could be the reason for it is, however, is unknown to most.'[1]

The alarming news referred to a survey conducted by market research institute GfK Health-Care from Nürnberg: 711 men between 45 and 70 years of age were asked to respond to a questionnaire where, by ticking appropriate boxes, they expressed how they were feeling. The paper did not reveal who commissioned and sponsored the publication of such alarming results – pharmaceutical company Dr Kade/Besins from Berlin.[2]

Around the same time, Jenapharm also jumped onto the male scourge bandwagon. In a study it says, 'Neither man himself, nor society wants to acknowledge that man also experiences a climacteric transition'. Elsewhere, the firm warns, 'A recurrent cause for the drop in performance over 40 is the age-related decrease in the hormone testosterone.'

It is no accident, though, that Kade/Besins and Jenapharm are so accommodating and understanding towards the male menopause. Since the spring of 2003, they have a product on the market, which is allegedly able to renovate the ruined male: a new gel enriched with testosterone, the hormone that turns boys into men.

Selling medical therapies is the pharmaceutical industry's business. In the case of testosterone deficiency the disease and the product are sold together. The 'hormone firms' are mobilising opinion research institutes, advertising agencies, PR enterprises, medical professors and journalists to publicise the male menopause as a serious and common disease

But does this disease really exist? The testosterone level doubtlessly decreases during a man's lifespan – but until now, physicians regarded this as a result of ageing. Testosterone is the most important male sex hormone (androgen) in humans. Chemically, testosterone is produced from cholesterol. This happens in the adrenal gland, but most importantly in the testicles.

After a man's fortieth birthday, his testosterone level drops every year by around 1 per cent. This is caused by a diminished functioning of the Leydig's cells in the testicles and an altered secretion of the luteinising hormone that stimulates the Leydig's cells.

The 1 per cent decrease in testosterone concentration, however, is based on estimates, since scientists compared hormone values of a number of young and older men. But because personal testosterone values are different between individuals, the procedure lacks precision.

It would be more precise to record the hormone profile of the same men over several decades, only very few such longitudinal studies have been carried out. In a small survey, the New Mexico ageing process study, hormonal changes in older men (61 to 87 years) were observed. The average decrease amounted to 110 nanograms per decilitre of blood over a decade. This decrease is so minimal that it might not appear significant at all, particularly when the body weight of the individuals is taken into account.[3]

In the spring of 2003, this natural drop was reinterpreted, at press conferences, in patient advice books, doctors' brochures and advertisements, as something pathological. Ageing male syndrome, virile climacteric, testosterone deficiency syndrome, age-related hypogonadism, andropause, Padam ('partial androgen-deficiency of ageing men') – old men's new sufferings were denoted by many names.

Heiner Mönig, endocrinologist at the University of Kiel, suspects, 'There are attempts to attach the stigma of disease to the physiological deterioration of the male gonads.'

The hormone in a tube could improve the well-being, love life, bone density and muscle strength of menopausal men, counter two firms that produce it. Their identical products are sold under the labels Androtop Gel (Kade/Besins) and Testogel (Jenapharm). The gels should be applied every morning to stomach or shoulders. For a month – depending on the dosage – one pack costs more than 65 Euros.

The synthetically produced hormone is not new, but the method of application is. The 1960s testosterone pills were a flop; 80 per cent of hormones taken orally are broken down by the liver – a biochemical tour de force, which is not good for the detox organ.

Also, the formerly very common method of injecting hormones supplied the body too unevenly. During the first hours and days, the circulation is flooded and towards the end of the three-week injection interval, the sex hormone circulates only sparsely. This hormonal roller coaster leads to abrupt mood swings; libido and physical strength also rise and fall.

Testosterone plasters also have their downside. They are best stuck directly onto the scrotum, because the scrotal skin is forty times more permeable than other body regions. Before this, the scrotum has to be carefully shaven, a procedure that most men find troublesome. The plaster may rustle and feel uncomfortable.

By contrast, the new hormone gel is easily applied to skin allowing the testosterone molecules to penetrate the body. The gel is a beneficent medicament for men with real hormone deficiency. Among them are castrates, eunuchs or men with Klinefelter's syndrome, a genetic disease whereby a man carries an additional x-chromosome.

Another category of patients has had their scrotums destroyed by viral inflammation, tumour or accident. The affected individuals have infantile sexual organs and accumulate fat in the abdominal region. Other typical traits in such cases include delicate, fair skin, a high-pitched voice, lack of facial and body hair, as well as underdeveloped muscles. In these patients with 'hypogonadism', artificially supplied testosterone stimulates the reappearance of male characteristics, which is why it is licensed as a drug for their cases.

But only a few men suffer from this disease. In Germany, there are, for example, nationwide fewer than 80,000 men with Klinefelter's syndrome – this figure is too small to be described as a testosterone-bestseller. However, more than 12 million men between the age of 50 and 80 live in Germany.

This is the point where medicine and marketing go their separate ways. At a strategic meeting at Kade/Besins in August 2002, a presenter stated, 'Androtop Gel will only be successful if demand for it is created.'[4] That is why the firm propagates testosterone now as some kind of antidote against ageing. 'Age in years: 58. Age in feeling: 48' is written on the cover of freshly printed patient brochures. Inside one can read about the many age-related problems 'you do not have to put up with any more'.[5]

Jenapharm blows the 'testosterone deficiency syndrome' out of all proportion by turning it into a public disease: 'Epidemiological estimates assume that at least 2.8 million people in Germany are affected.'[6] The American National Institute on Aging goes as far as to announce in its report that – depending on how the alleged deficiency is defined – up to '50 per cent of older men could be considered' for testosterone replacement therapy.[7]

Pharmaceutical concerns and physicians groups have already, once before, mastered the tricky business of turning a healthy section of the population into hormone-deficient creatures. In Germany, one in four women over 40 takes oestrogen preparations.

It is now men's turn. At the Kade/Besins meeting in August 2002, the picture of an older woman was presented. 'Hormones helped me to fight nervousness, hot flushes and listlessness', advertising experts prompt her to say. 'I wish this were available for my husband too.'

Nevertheless, the Federal Institute for Drugs and Medicinal Products in Bonn would not license the use of testosterone gels for anything like a male menopause. It warns that the gel should be used only in cases of 'proven hypogonadism, i.e. diminution of functional activity in the testes'. In spite of this, there is nothing to stand in the way of prescriptions on a massive scale. For, because of the freedom of therapy, every doctor is allowed to prescribe any already licensed drug beyond its actual indication.

The support of medical expert societies is extremely beneficial for market expansion. Therefore, it was very timely for the industry that in the summer of 2000 twelve German professors of urology and endocrinology described the 'ageing-man' syndrome for the first time in a 'consensus paper'.[8]

Hermann Behre, a member of the study group and professor of andrology at the University of Halle, Germany, is now giving well-paid lectures for the testosterone firms. In January he represented Kade/Besins and in March Jenapharm, praising the advantages of the hormone gel at press conferences.

In the United States also, the testosterone campaign attracted doctors who were willing to serve its cause. An association of American endocrinology researchers, the renowned Endocrine Society, dedicated in April 2000 a whole conference in Beverly Hills, California to the topic of andropause – six weeks before the gel was launched onto the US market.

At the conference, the endocrinologists who gathered came up with contradictory advice. It is true, they admitted, that the benefit of testosterone supply had not been proven. Nonetheless, they advised that the hormone level of all men over 50 be measured. Moreover, they defined a threshold of 10.4 nanomol of testosterone per litre of blood. If the level falls below this value, said the doctors, then the patient would 'probably benefit from treatment'.

Jerome Groopman from Harvard Medical School might not doubt that the physicians passed judgement with good intentions. But it's also the case, he said, that 'a Unimed/Solvay educational grant was the sole source of funding for the Beverly Hills conference'. The firm Unimed – daughter firm of Belgian Solvay and distributor of the testosterone gel in the United States – had even propositioned several members. In total, thirteen doctors were sitting on the andropause committee – at least nine of them had, according to the *New Yorker*, financial connections to the pharmaceutical company.[9]

In comparison with their US colleagues, the German medical professors have set the threshold in their consensus paper even higher: at twelve. Anyone below this value is accordingly suffering from testosterone deficiency. Overnight, 20 per cent of 60 year olds and 35 per cent of those over 80 were thereby declared ill.[10]

This threshold was selected in a completely arbitrary way, says Frankfurt urologist Gerd Ludwig, who ironically enough contributed to the rendering of the consensus paper. The values were those of young men and had simply been applied to members of the more mature generation. 'Whether such a minimum threshold is applicable to the older man at all, is very questionable', says Ludwig. Many older men had testosterone levels 'of five, six or eight nanomol and did not display any symptoms at all'.[11]

In companies' advertising campaigns, the controversial threshold value has become a scientific expert opinion. Jenapharm generously estimates that 'approximately every third man over the age of 55' had values below the magical twelve and then announces to journalists, 'In these cases, clinicians talk about hypogonadism, a disease.'[12]

Are man's best years then a cause for medicine? Scientifically, 'the male menopause' is not exactly a proven fact: 80-year-old men, for example, have on average still half as much freely available testosterone in their blood as a 30 year old and are able to father children. Overall, a general correlation between testosterone values in older age and medical conditions has not been established. In spite of lower values, many men are doing splendidly, whereas others have a hormone high but feel worn out.

Physician William Crowley from Massachusetts General Hospital set out a couple of years ago in search of the andropause. In order to study hypogonadism, he first looked for a definition to determine what a normal testosterone level actually was. To do so, the doctor took a few drops of blood every ten minutes over a period of twenty-four hours from healthy young men. In addition, the test persons were examined like breeding stallions at an auction. The size of their testicles, body hair pattern, erection capacity, ejaculated sperm count, bone density, muscle mass and function of pituitary gland were measured and evaluated by doctors. These values were all within the normal range. Only the testosterone levels made the researchers curious: 15 per cent of the healthy men had values way below the range which American physicians had formerly defined as normal.[13]

The experiment shows that based on blood values alone, it is not possible to diagnose hormone deficiency. Equally important is the number and condition of receptors – that is the docking stations – for testosterone in the body. Only when it docks with a receptor, can testosterone unleash its anabolic power. When these receptors are defective or unavailable, even the highest testosterone level has no effect. Conversely, those with particularly effective receptors will be able to manage with a little less testosterone.

In the same person, hormone values may fluctuate within relatively short periods of time. Physical activity, for example, influences the level. Half an hour of jogging pushes the testosterone level up by a third, whereas stress is generally known to diminish the amount of sex hormones.

Such fluctuations still cannot be explained to endocrinologists' satisfaction. When William Crowley later examined the men who had had low levels, he found that their levels were much higher. This means for laboratory diagnosis that low measured values do not necessarily signal hormone deficiency. Moreover, present measuring technology is unreliable. If identical blood samples are measured with the methods of different producers, often completely different values crop up.

After elaborate consultations, a committee of the American National Institute on Aging published a report in 2001 according to which the whole concept of andropause is questionable. 'The evidence for associations of measures of serum testosterone with health outcomes are inconsistent and inconclusive.'[14] The International Society for the Study of the Aging Male gives warnings as well. Because of the inconclusive data situation it was 'somewhat premature' to provide guidelines for the therapy of andropause.[15]

The marketeers, however, continue to praise testosterone as a possible elixir against loss of sexual appetite, bad temper, slack muscles, hot flushes and brittle bones. Yet most of the statements are based on experiments with a modest sample of 227 men, and often with only 7 or 11 men.

When medical doctors from the University of Pennsylvania in Philadelphia had a closer look, the claimed effect of testosterone on bone density vanished. Over a three-year period, the researchers supplied 108 men over 65 with the hormone. Compared with a test group that had received a placebo, there was no measurable difference.[16]

Even if testosterone is 'really beneficial for life quality is not yet proven', urologist Wolfgang Weidner from Gießen reminds us. Up to now, the companies have economised on the funding for necessary studies – or they have preferred to put it towards their advertising campaigns. In the spring of 2003, pharmaceutical consultants travelled the country to acquaint the medical profession with the new male syndrome.

Discreetly the hormone gel is made palatable to doctors as a 'wellness-drug' too. Thus, the Kade/Besins firm suggests prescribing the gel, should the occasion arise, beyond the threshold value as well. In a glossy brochure ('guidelines for the physician'), the pharmaceutical company explains to the general practitioner how this works: 'If laboratory values are within the normal range, a proposal for privately paid treatment could be made to the patient.'[17]

However, anyone who has enough endogenous testosterone at his disposal will not experience any additional virility boost at all through the extra dose of hormone. In the case of normal testosterone levels, most of the receptors are already occupied. Additional molecules cannot dock anywhere and disappear as if in a puff of smoke. Clinicians compare this effect to a car running on a half-empty tank. The vehicle will not drive any faster if it is filled up.

Having said that, a multitude of side effects threatens the top-up user. Long-term treatment with testosterone can alter the fat metabolism and possibly raise the risk of cardiac infarct. Damage to the liver may also occur, which is why patients with already weakened organs should be excluded from treatment. Moreover, blood formation is cranked up. True, doctors want to get rid of anaemia in older age, but this may well backfire: thrombosis or life-threatening embolisms might be triggered.

When the body receives more testosterone than necessary from external sources, it can reduce its own production – the testicles shrivel. In addition, the spermatozoa do not tolerate the hormone profusion well and consequently waste away – the capacity to procreate decreases. When young people are supplied with additional hormone, bone growth may stop prematurely – the young person remains a squirt. Finally, there is the threat of a bizarre overdose reaction: the body transforms too much testosterone into the female sex hormone oestrogen – the male users grow female breasts, a phenomenon called 'gynaecomasty'.

If women come into contact with the testosterone gel, they are also threatened by severe side effects. Only around 10 per cent of the masculinity hormone contained in the gel actually penetrates the body. Unsuspecting women rubbing up against the skin of their freshly gelled partners not only might find their pleasure feeling increased, but also might be blessed with beard growth, a deeper voice, acne or hair loss.

For these reasons, the producers of the gel warn people to take precautionary measures. After gelling the abdomen, hands should be washed with soap and a T-shirt should be put on for safety. In the United States, the Federal Drug Agency warned when licensing the treatment that pregnant women should keep their distance from gelled men because testosterone could harm the unborn child.

The biggest danger is probably the one that threatens the male prostate gland. Animal experiments have shown that testosterone may induce prostate cancer. Many experts suspect such a correlation exists for humans as well – accordingly the synthetic hormone would waken dormant cancer seats. In at least one-third of 60-year-old men and in every second man over 70 these are lurking in the prostate.

Even a study conducted by the producer revealed an effect on the prostate gland. Almost 20 per cent of long-term users, who had treated themselves to 100 milligrams every morning, complained about acute prostate problems. In one of the test persons, doctors discovered a newly developed prostate cancer; three others discontinued the hormone treatment because of troubles with the prostate gland.[18]

The US government planned a long-term study to solve the mystery of the andropause. The Department of Veterans Affairs and the National Institute on Aging wanted to spend $110 million on a six-year medical trial with 6,000 men across forty medical centres. The mammoth project, however, was brought to a halt in June 2002 shortly before the scheduled start date. Physicians did not want to expose test persons to the possible risks of testosterone.[19]

But even without studies about long-term risks, doctors will still prescribe the masculinity hormone – as did physicians who some decades ago arbitrarily propagated hormone replacement for women. John McKinlay from the New England Research Institute near Boston fears:

We are about to repeat that debacle. We have the slimmest evidence on testosterone replacement. Five men here, ten men there. Six rats and a partridge in a pear tree. The physiology is not there but the industry, the industry is there.

For ten years, the endocrinologist has been measuring the hormone level of 2,000 men between 39 and 70 years of age. McKinlay's conclusion: 'Call it what you like – andropause, viropause, bullshit – there is no evidence, epidemiological, scientific or clinical, to support its existence. The whole notion of the andropause is the medicalisation of normal aging.'[20]

Why eunuchs live longer

If testosterone is supposed to help against the loathed ageing process, then it is perhaps only because it shortens the lifespan considerably. This is at least what long-term studies comparing castrated and unscathed men suggest. Castrated men, who have had to manage without testicles and thereby without testosterone, live on average fifteen years longer than their intact counterparts. And the earlier the castration was executed, the more effective was its life-prolonging effect.

The comparatively early decease of normal men was caused by their endogenous testosterone, believes biologist Ian Owens from Imperial College London. In fact, the masculinity hormone weakens the body's immune reaction. It probably reduces energy supply to the immune system so that the man is able to use his strength for other activities. The testosterone effect was confirmed by a comparative study involving castrates. Infectious diseases – not violence or accidents – were to blame for the elevated death rate of normal men.[21]

Researchers therefore explain the early death of the stronger sex by testosterone. In western countries, men die on average seven years earlier than women. Men die more often in car accidents and are more often victims of homicide and suicide; they are more often infected by AIDS and consume more drugs than women.

However, if we disregard these risky lifestyle deaths, there remains a difference in life expectancy. Apparently, men offer bacteria and parasites a better attack surface than women. On the one hand, the male body is simply bigger than the female. On the other hand, man produces large quantities of a substance that undermines his immunity: testosterone.[22]

The fairy-tale of the fountain of youth

The quest for eternal youth is as old as humankind itself. The business of alchemists in the Middle Ages flourished particularly brilliantly because gold was regarded the most potent elixir for longevity. Nowadays, some doctors, natural scientists and dubious entrepreneurs have slipped into the role of quacks. In the guise of an 'anti-ageing-medicine', they are bombarding the public with half-truths to an unprecedented extent. Ageing and its accompanying phenomena are portrayed as diseases to be eliminated.

'Already at the age of fifty, our bodies produce only a third of the original hormone amount – health troubles are pre-programmed', announces for example the German Society for Anti-Ageing Medicine (headquarters in Munich). In this society, 600 members have united forces to study how the ageing process might be postponed, halted or even reversed. On a 'fact sheet', the anti-ageing doctors suggest along-side testosterone and oestrogen also other hormones to fight against the vanishing of youth:

- Administering DHEA (Dehydroepiandrosterone) increases libido and well-being. It lowers the cholesterol level, aids breakdown of fat tissues and improves the ability to concentrate.
- According to the brochure, giving melatonin protects against oxygen radicals, improves the immune system and dispels depressive moods.
- Consumption of growth hormones, finally, is supposed to stimulate cell regeneration, improve the tone of connective tissue, increase libido and strengthen the immune system.

It all sounds plausible – yet it is not quite true. No hormone preparations, no vitamins, no anti-oxidants, no surgery, not even any lifestyle changes are demonstrably able to influence the ageing process.

This regrettable, but biologically true conclusion was drawn in 2002 by Jay Olshansky from the University of Illinois in Chicago together with other leading ageing researchers of the United States. The fifty-one scientists urge the public not to heed the false promises of the fountain of youth industry: 'The people should know that no currently marketed intervention – none – has yet been proved to slow, stop or reverse human aging, and some can be downright dangerous.' Neither in animals nor in humans have the researchers so far identified a yard-stick for physical decay – the hands on the clock of ageing have not yet been discovered. But without reliable reference points the anti-ageing prophets cannot tell at all whether their acts have any effect.[23]

Once the engine of life switches on, it runs inevitably towards its own destruction. Slipped discs, broken hipbones, wrinkles, cataracts, haemorrhoids, varicose veins, but also altered proteins and mutated genes are the expression of the unpleasant yet natural change. In the course of decades accidental damage accumulates in the big and small building blocks of the body – ageing is nothing else. Youth repair mechanisms work against the ever present decay, it is true, but at some stage, they just cannot handle the defects any more – an inevitable tragedy.

Cells, tissues and organs work only in a restricted way – age reveals its face: muscles and bones lose their mass, eyesight and hearing weaken, skin wrinkles, reaction time decreases. In addition, the person becomes more susceptible to diseases, such as heart diseases, Alzheimer's, cancer or stroke. The researches into ageing led by Jay Olshansky maintain that these diseases are

> age-related conditions . . . superimposed on aging, not equivalent to it. Therefore, even if science could eliminate today's leading killers of older individuals, aging would continue to occur, ensuring that different maladies would take their place. In addition, it would guarantee that one crucial body component or another – say the cardiovascular system – would eventually experience a catastrophic failure.[24]

Since 1840, life expectancy in industrial nations has increased steadily, every year by three months. Scientists from the Max Planck Institute for Demographic Research in Rostock assume that the biological age barrier has not yet been reached. In the year 2060, the average life expectancy could theoretically be one hundred years.[25] People in rich countries do not live longer, however, because they age differently but because they live differently. Welfare, medicaments, nutrition and particularly hygiene play a role.

Nonetheless, genes which determine life expectancy do not exist. Evolution favours genes which give an advantage for procreation and consequently for transmission of genetic material. What happens to a human being after the phase of procreation and rearing children is no longer subject to the selective mechanisms of evolution. It is true that a number of hereditary dispositions influence ageing, but this happens only by indirect effects – an 'ageing gene' does not exist. That humans have a life expectancy of seven and more decades is, in

the light of evolution, purely accidental. This has dramatic consequences for medicine, the ageing researchers remind us: 'The lack of
a specific genetic program for aging and death means that there is
no quick fixes that will permit us to treat aging as if it were a disease'.

Even with exercise and healthy nutrition, we cannot change the
destiny of ageing. Sport and reasonable eating habits can help us
avoid diseases. This way we can harness a healthier and longer life –
but we cannot put off ageing itself.

9 Whenever you want it

The penis does not at all obey the orders of his master.

Leonardo da Vinci

Up it goes. At least for the 17 million plus men worldwide who, since 1998, have experienced the blue miracle: Viagra. The octagonal pill with sky-blue coating works better against impotence than any other method before it. Every second, the potency drug is taken by four men somewhere in the world. The temptation is very real: for the first time erection disorders can be managed conveniently with a pill; the only thing one has to remember is to take it on time, around half an hour before the planned act.

'My wife said I was like Tarzan', remembers the 62-year-old Alfred Pariser from Los Angeles, one of the very first men who had the pleasure of experiencing the arousing drug. The now happy man had been impotent since doctors removed the tumorous prostate from his lower abdomen. As a participant in a clinical trial, Pariser took Viagra – and he regained his erection.

However, Viagra – and its new competitors Cialis from US firm Lilly Icos and Levitra from the house of Bayer – are much more than chemical penis erectors. These medications have changed the world. The pornographic industry, just to mention one example, has experienced a real revolution. Long gone are the times when male leads needed length breaks or a stand-in for close-ups. 'Nowadays, the shooting is often only interrupted for a make-up touch-up, a visit to the toilet or a coffee break', reports the Germany press agency dpa from San Fernando, California, stronghold of the American porn industry.

And scholars of anatomy owe the potency pill insights that previously seemed impossible. It was not until Viagra that men finally managed, inside the uncomfortable tube of a computer tomograph

(measuring 50 centimetres in diameter), to penetrate women and
remain motionless at the summit of lust for 12 seconds. The truly
sharp pictures taken of the test persons' lower abdomen, meanwhile,
did satisfy an old question: how precisely do men and women inter-
connect? The answer is thanks to an astonishing kink of nature. The
penis describes a curve upwards and fits into the vagina like a boom-
erang, announced researchers from the University of Groningen.[1]

In addition, Viagra expands the repertoire of reproductive medicine.
Some men simply cannot withstand the pressure of expectations when
it comes to those intimate meetings that mainly serve the purpose of
reproduction. 'They feel like breeding bulls', explains a urologist from
the University of Gießen, 'Then I give them a Viagra tablet and things
are okay.'

Viagra, the summit of present pharmaceutical research, has changed
the world. The pill has changed people's sex lives, at least as far as the
male half of the population is concerned, into a medical need, which
everybody can obtain per prescription. Some gentlemen are not up to
this ruse, though. Since Viagra was introduced in 1998, at least thirty
consumers in Germany alone have remained 'eternally stiff', as the
Berlin daily *taz* smugly put it. Worldwide there have been more than
600 fatalities to date. Particularly wild was Sani Abacha's death,
once a military dictator in Nigeria. The 54-year-old general, pumped
full of Viagra, died on 8 June 1998, at the summit of an orgy with
three Indian prostitutes.

The industry does not find any of this funny; for many millions of
impotent men this is serious business. Until the beginning of 2003
Viagra dominated the market. In the year 2001 it realised a turnover
amounting to one and a half billion dollars; the manufacturer Pfizer
became the world's biggest pharmaceutical company.

The grandiose success story affected the whole pharmaceutical
industry like some kind of research-Viagra: the first potency pill in
1998 might have left humankind windswept. In the mean time, however, a whirlwind has been building on the horizon. At least twenty
new sex substances for men are undergoing testing and licensing
phases at the laboratories of pill producers. Since 2003, the first successor products have been hitting the market. They are substances which,
like their famous model Viagra, directly affect the corpus cavernosum
of the penis, but which have supposedly a more thorough, faster and
longer effect.[2]

American pharmaceutical corporation Lilly Icos is offering an
almond-shaped pill called Cialis with particularly long-lived effect; it
may provide a man with uplifting support through a whole weekend.

As for the German Bayer enterprise, its group of twenty biologists and chemists developed, in the record time of only two years, a substance astonishingly similar to Viagra's active agent, yet supposedly even more effective. Under the name of Levitra, Bayer, together with the pharmaceutical giant GlaxoSmithKline, is marketing the apricot-coloured potency pill around the world. They all want to make profit on the myth that only a perfect erection is within the normal bounds.

Sex as compulsory exercise

The fuss about Viagra and the like makes the up until now lacklustre field of urology positively glitter. Once specialising in bladder stones, kidney aches and prostate troubles, the discipline is now in its heyday thanks to the subject of sex.

Ahead of the field is Irwin Goldstein, a urologist, who holds a chair for sexual medicine at Boston University – a department of which there exists only one even in the United States. In collaboration with his colleagues, Goldstein freed the phenomenon of impotence from its psycho-image in the mid 1980s. Since then the absence of male stiffness is no longer treated on the couch – but at the laboratory.

'Not to discount psychological aspects', announces Goldstein, 'but at a certain point all sex is mechanical. The man needs a sufficient axial rigidity so his penis can penetrate through labia.'

Consequently, the urologist wants to erect the limp organ in a way similar to what an astronaut would do to get his defective space ship underway again. 'I am an engineer', continues Goldstein, who did in fact collaborate with Boston University's Department of Aerospace Engineering in formulating his theories to overcome erection weakness, 'and I can apply the principles of hydraulics to these problems.'[3]

Once, medical doctors preached public chastity and morality. In the 1950s, the only 'normal' thing was conventional marital intercourse. Up to the beginning of the Second World War in 1939, young women who were pregnant, but not married, could be sent to a lunatic asylum, for an undetermined length of time. Sexual variants fell to the competence of psychiatrists. In the first edition of the *Diagnostic and Statistical Manual of Mental Disorders* from 1952, homosexuality was described as a distinct and treatable disease. Affected persons would be castrated or treated with hormones.

Now, once again biomechanics, pharmacologists and physicians take over people's sex life – but this time in a very different way. Nowadays they prescribe them a medicine where regular sex is part of health – no matter if people feel like it or not. 'Relatively recently, the imperative was for restraint and moderation in sexual matters; now it is for more and better sexual gratification', contemplate British health researchers Graham Hart and Kaye Wellings Abstinence is now regarded 'the new deviance' – and therefore becomes a case for disease mongering.[4]

Urologist Hartmut Porst is among the elite of new sex doctors. His surgery at Neue Jungfernstieg in Hamburg is flourishing; its database contains the names of hundreds of limp men from all over Germany. With them as guinea pigs, Porst is conducting the highest number of studies worldwide on the effectiveness and safety of potency drugs and pleasure pills. Industry researchers from all around the globe entrust the German doctor with their latest creations for inspection.

On a February day in 2002, Porst's recruits ingest an experimental active agent from a Japanese company; the substance is supposed to kindle lust directly in their brains. The fourteen test subjects are lying naked in bed watching porn videos. After around 30 minutes, the test substance starts to kick in – the sex doctor makes his round. Is anything stirring yet? Expectantly he pulls off the lemon-yellow blanket covering his 58-year-old patient Johannes I. The skinny man, wearing only socks, smiles in embarrassment. 'There you are', mutters Porst, writes a remark in the patient's folder and hurries to see the next test person. At the end of his round, he seems content: 'I've seen some really good erections.'

Doubtlessly, Porst's inspection is not to everybody's taste. Nevertheless, it is necessary for the search for new sex pills. 'There is almost no other field of medicine where there is so much happening as in the development of new drugs against sexual disorders', explains Hartmut Porst. 'We are currently experiencing the second sexual revolution.'

Viagra for the ladies

It wasn't the dissatisfied men who instigated the coup. Pharmaceutical researchers and marketing people were the ones who set the stage for sexual frustration to make its appearance as a widespread and treatable phenomenon. Moreover, all of a sudden, they claim to have discovered that sexual frigidity is also severely rampant among women: 43 per cent of adult women are supposedly suffering from it. Scepticism seems more than desirable here – the remarkably high number is for the industry a billion dollar equation.

'The necessity to find a remedy for the lack of female libido is enormous', claims American drug researcher Perry Molinoff. He is experimenting with the substance 'PT-141', which is supposed to directly affect the sex centre in the human brain. Oysters, champagne, vibrator and candlelight will soon be out of fashion, rejoices Molinoff, 'PT-141 is the first known substance that seems to kindle female desire.'

Through his pharmaceutical firm Palatin Technologies in Edison, New Jersey, Molinoff wants to launch the alleged aphrodisiac today rather than tomorrow: as a nasal spray for foreplay. Tests on four rhesus monkeys and the first clinical trials on sixteen women, who sprayed PT-141 into each nostril, went satisfactorily well, assures Molinoff. The ladies, dosed with PT-141, watched erotic videos while small devices measured the blood flow through their vaginas. In comparison with sixteen women who had taken a nasal spray without active agent, more blood did indeed gush through the tissues of female PT-141 users.

PT-141 has an effect similar to the hormone melanotropin that occurs naturally in the human brain. Among its various tasks, it encourages tanning when the skin is exposed to ultra-violet rays. It was for precisely this reason that researchers at the Health Science Center at the University of Arizona noticed PT-141. They had given the substance as a suntan application to very pale men to encourage their pigmentation.

Indeed, the men were soon pleased with their deep tan and also with the astonishing side effects: mighty erections. One of the researchers who had used the application on his skin out of pure curiosity wandered about with a stiff penis for eight hours. No wonder the industry soon got interested. The suntan application had apparently aroused the test persons' desire from brain downwards. 'We probably had a psychogenic response setting up a cascade of responses down the spinal column to give a very natural, normal erectile response', explains pharmacologist Mac Hadley from the University of Arizona.[5]

However, if PT-141 really stimulates sexual appetite, were the longed-for sex pills not a danger to humanity? Perry Molinoff reassures, 'As a nasal spray it does not affect the brain for very long. And one would only sniff it before an imminent sexual activity.' Through mucous membrane and blood vessels, PT-141 reaches the brain within seconds. This way of administering the substance was carefully chosen, explains Molinoff: 'A pill could be dropped secretly into a woman's drink and make her love-crazed.'

Researchers at industry leader Pfizer are also very keen. They are examining whether their classic Viagra could perhaps also have an effect on women who are difficult to arouse. Therefore, Pfizer conducted secret tests with its potency pill on English women – without any real success, however. Throughout the industry, companies are testing at least a dozen preparations in clinical trials – various pills and creams gels and nasal sprays that are supposed to arouse female desire.

No doubt about it. Pharmaceutical researchers dream of restaging the gigantic economic success of the men's Viagra pills in the women's world. Preparation is underway at breakneck speed – and by no means just in the laboratory. What the pill manufacturers need foremost in order to market their products is a clearly defined medical picture; ideally, a syndrome that is determinable by specific characteristics.

Discovery of the lustless women

A long time ago, pharmaceutical companies set to work. Over several years they have regularly sponsored conferences and meetings where the outlines of precisely such a disease began to emerge. The condition was christened 'female sexual dysfunction'. Once again, the finding comes at just the right moment for the industry, particularly since it has allegedly affected almost half of the female population.

The epidemic spread of this 'lustlessness' syndrome was, however, exposed as a purely artificial construct. The 'making of female sexual dysfunction is the freshest, clearest example for the corporate sponsored creation of a disease', reports Ray Moynihan in the *British Medical Journal*:

> A cohort of researchers with close ties to drug companies are working with colleagues in the pharmaceutical industry to develop and define a new category of human illness at meetings heavily sponsored by companies racing to develop new drugs.[6]

Accordingly, the female condition was established in 1997 during a 'sex conference' held at a hotel in Cape Cod, Massachusetts. At a follow-up meeting in Boston that October, the alleged 'no sex thank you' syndrome was defined more precisely – behind closed doors and sponsored by pharmaceutical companies. Of the nineteen authors, who later published the results of what seemed like a conspiracy meeting, eighteen had connections to the industry. Their consensus paper was in turn financially supported by eight companies. Finally, the physicians founded a 'Female Sexual Function Forum'. It organised conferences in Boston, which were sponsored by more than twenty pharmaceutical companies. Co-organiser of these meetings was none other than Irwin Goldstein, the US urologist, who wants to repair sexual disorders like a mechanic. His close ties to the industry seem almost too intimate. As a consultant and lecturer he works, according to his own account, 'for virtually every pharmaceutical company'. In December 2002, the tireless Goldstein entered the ring at a 'potency symposium' in Hamburg, sponsored by the Levitra manufacturer Bayer and by GlaxoSmithKline.[7]

Female sexual dysfunction had reached its first heights in the year 1999, when the medical journal *JAMA* published the result of a survey on the topic: 43 per cent of all women aged between 18 and 59 complained about their unsatisfying love life – a gigantic pool of female patients. Once the figure had seen the light of day, it quickly went the rounds; most of the media picked up on it and uncritically publicised it further.[8]

It emerged later on, however, that two of the four study authors had ties to the sex pill concern Pfizer. What was even graver was that the methods of the researchers, sociologists from the University of Chicago, were extremely dubious. They extracted their 43 per cent claim, which was to have such a magnitude of consequences, from a mass of old data that had been collected seven years earlier. At that time, 1,500 women had been asked about their sex lives during the previous year, namely whether they had felt for more than two months one of seven symptoms such as no desire for sex, fear of failure in bed or vaginal dryness. Anyone who answered 'yes' to at least one of the questions was labelled by the sociologists as a person with a sexual dysfunction. In this way, problems of the healthy metamorphose into conditions of the sick.

Common sense rebels against such an approach. The desire for sex is undoubtedly closely linked to stress, tiredness and moods in a relationship. Not feeling sexual desire is, in certain life situations, normal and healthy. John Bancroft, sex researcher and director of the Kinsey Institute at Indiana University, warns about a fatal development. To depict sexual problems as functional disorders holds the danger, says Bancroft, that 'it is likely to encourage doctors to prescribe drugs to change sexual function when the attention should be paid to other aspects of the woman's life'.

At least this critique was not completely ignored. The Chicago sociologists have backed off. Many women from the 43 per cent group were 'perfectly normal', Edward Laumann, the researcher in charge, now admits. Many of their problems, he adds – and we listen amazed – would 'arise out of perfectly reasonable responses of the human organism to challenges and stress'.

Nonetheless, should the often invoked pleasure pill for *her* hit the market, the female sexual dysfunction would, overnight, become a national disease. This is at least what the example of Viagra teaches us. Since Viagra's introduction, the diagnosis 'erectile dysfunction' is made much more often than formerly; in the United Kingdom for example three times more often.[9]

Average Joe turns into tireless lover

Certainly, many impotent men are seeing the doctor about their problems for the first time, because the doctor can finally help them. Among them are a great number of men who have serious conditions – men who have had prostate operations, diabetics, kidney disease sufferers, high blood pressure patients and arteriosclerosis sufferers. On the other hand, Viagra has also changed sexual behaviour. Thanks to the potency pill, healthy men want to mutate into untiring lovers. In view of the chemical alternative, whatever 'degree of lust' nature has bestowed on them seems in their view to be crying out for improvement. British health researchers Graham Hart and Kaye Wellings have established that many 'who once thought their low libido was "normal" and acceptable now feel dissatisfied with their sexual lives'.[10]

Potency pill producers add fuel to the fire of such male longings. On the one hand, they seek to attract new customers with enlightening advertisements on impotence – pardon, erectile dysfunction. Or with questionnaires, which men may fill out discreetly on the Internet. 'Test yourself', the Lilly firm coos, 'and discuss the result with your doctor'.[11]

On the other hand, companies tirelessly portray impotence as a widespread yet threatening condition. 'Erectile disorders are a serious and common health condition: approximately 50 per cent of men between the age of 40 and 70 are affected', claims Pfizer.[12] This generalisation is misleading. The Massachusetts Male Aging Study involving 1,300 men has shown that only 10 per cent had complete erectile weakness. In 25 per cent of the cases, the dysfunction was 'moderate', and in 17 per cent only 'minimal'.

Other surveys that produced even lower impotence figures are unlikely to reach the spotlight. A survey of 4,500 German men between 30 and 80 years of age, the Cologne Male Survey, showed 19.2 per cent of surveyed men with an average age of 52 have erectile calm. And according to a study from Italy, only 2 per cent of men under 39 complain that will alone was sometimes not enough. It is also clear that the frequency of impotence increases with age.[13]

In Pfizer's advertisements, however, young and healthy men appear more and more often – obviously in the search of a fresh market. In early adverts American ex-senator Bob Dole described himself at the age of 74 as lacking in potency. At the beginning of 2002, Pfizer turned towards a younger target group and chose 43-year-old, popular American racing driver Mark Martin for its advertising. On the bonnet of his roaring Ford Taurus and on his overall as well, the magic word 'Viagra' can now be admired. In a press advert the company also adopts a snappy tone. A handsome man around 40 asks cockily,'Think you're too young for Viagra?'[14]

That fit young men want to take the potency enhancers to increase their erectile ability seems par for the course. 'Anything that has to do with sex inevitably relates to lifestyle', states urologist Hartmut Porst from Hamburg. There is no problem in getting your hands on the remedy, which should, strictly speaking, be dispensed on prescription. Viagra and the like can be ordered – without visiting a doctor – over the Internet. 'That the healthy take a drug to have a better erection', says Porst, 'is something that cannot be prevented.'

No wonder then that marketing experts display a confident attitude. In Germany, the turnover of potency remedies – up until the beginning of 2003 realised almost exclusively by Viagra – amounted to 50 million Euros per year. Because of the new competitor products Cialis and Levitra – as well as their advertising campaigns – the sales are expected to rise tremendously to 150 or 200 million Euros per year, so market researchers estimate.

At the same time, there is increasing pressure on German health insurance schemes to pay for the costs of potency drugs. In Stuttgart a 72-year-old pensioner with erectile problems brought his case before the social welfare court after his health insurer refused to pay for Viagra. In December 2001 the social welfare court of Baden-Württemberg passed a judgment that said the man was in the right. Diabetic civil servants also receive Viagra at the state's expense. And so the Bavarian administrative court, in April 2003, set a new precedent. The plaintiff had referred to the fact that sexual activity is among the basic human needs enumerated by the WHO. The retired civil servant was suffering from erectile disorders because of diabetes and his doctor prescribed him Viagra. However, the health insurance for civil servants would not cover the expensive pill. The pensioner pursued a four-year law suit – and won. The precedent threatens health insurers with a bill of millions for sex by prescription.

Coitus at the expense of public health insurance would become even more likely if a new indication for the sex pills were to be found. This is precisely what some medics have on their minds. Viagra should not merely be a therapy for erectile disorders but should also help to main-tain penis health generally. Urologist Irwin Goldstein is a proponent here too. 'If you would like to be sexually active in five years' time, take a quarter of a pill a night', announced the sex professor at a conference in New York, sponsored by Pfizer. The daily Viagra dose prolongs the duration of nightly erections and maintains the function of lean muscle cells in the corpus cavernosum. At the present time, however, scientific proof justifying prophylactic treatment with Viagra is lacking.[15]

Sex therapist Leonore Tiefer from New York University described this last advance of the potency pharmacy as 'almost grotesque'.[16] The self-professed feminist is dreading a future when the sexes would meet in a drug-induced state of arousal. Geriatric affairs would risk potentially damaging and painful consequences. 'We're now going to have the 20-year-old vagina in the 60-year-old lady to go with the 20-year-old erection in the 60-year-old man', prophesises Tiefer. 'I'm not sure the genitalia can bear all that.'

A slim consolation remains. The new potency remedies and pleasure pills will lead indirectly to beautiful deaths: 'mors in coitu'. The penis, such a 'venerable symbol in itself' (so claims philosopher Friedrich Nietzsche), is in fact an important mirror of male health. If the precious bit is limp the owner may be at risk of cardiac infarct or stroke. If such a frail candidate suddenly has sex again, invigorated by potency drugs after years of abstinence, it could well be that he rises from the climax of pleasure to an even higher place – directly to heaven.

10 Destiny in our genes

The sequence is only the beginning . . .

J. Craig Venter

On 26 June 2000, the birth of homo geneticus was officially announced at the White House in Washington; the event resembled an imperial coronation, with incense, organ music and ceremonial trumpets. US President Bill Clinton and – via satellite from London – British Prime Minister Tony Blair appeared before the world audience, surrounded by glamorous dignitaries of science. Henceforth, we have a new map at our disposal, announced Clinton; without a doubt it is the most important and marvellous map that has ever been drawn by humankind. It holds the chance 'to understand the language in which god created life'.

He was of course referring to the human genome and the fact that the entire sequence of our chromosomes, consisting of 3 billion building blocks (pairs of bases), had almost completely been deciphered. Researchers had proposed the human genome project and been able to get it subsidised with billions of taxpayers' money, by promising politicians and citizens that the sequence would improve the health of humans. The DNA code was a starting point for developing new therapies for hereditary diseases and the many illnesses that are, in part, genetically conditioned.

On the day of the official decoding, promises of salvation were made with generosity. Clinton congratulated Blair saying that the life expectancy of his newly born son had risen on this day by twenty-five years. Over the forthcoming years, the US president prophesied cures for Alzheimer's, Parkinson's, diabetes and cancer. The deciphered genome would enhance life – for all citizens of this world.

The first products promising to fulfil that prophesy are now for sale. These gene tests for all supposedly enhance one's health prospects. ˈ ˈˈ ˈˈˈˈˈˈ , ˈˈˈˈˈˈˈˈ ˈˈˈˈˈˈˈˈ ˈˈˈˈˈˈˈˈ ˈˈˈ ˈˈˈˈˈˈˈˈ, ˈˈˈ ˈˈˈˈˈˈ to every person which nutrition and lifestyle would be suitable for him or her.' The firm Sciona developed the first gene test in the world to be available at the supermarket: 'You & Your Genes' is the name of the procedure, which examines nine genes and is said to bring a 'longer' and 'healthier life'. Customers are healthy people who believe in the promises of the lifestyle industry.

Sciona offers its genotype pattern pinpointing kit all over the world by telephone, on the Internet and since spring 2002 even in certain branches of the Body Shop in Britain. The worldwide cosmetics chain, which condemns animal testing and celebrates recycling, thereby paves the way to a brave new medicine. The 'radically new examination' of the genetic make-up, according to the Body Shop, would fulfil the promise of 'body and nutrition working together in harmony'. Gene test customers have to fill in a questionnaire about their eating, drinking and smoking habits; they are asked to place a special cotton bud on the inside of the cheek and rub it for a minute or so. Approximately 2,000 cells get stuck to the bud, which the customer then sends in a sealed tube to Sciona.

The firm has established itself at an industrial estate in the southern English town of Havant. The British Ministry for Trade and Industry has conferred upon the newly founded enterprise the 'Smart Award', a much sought-after research award. At the brand new laboratories, employees first extract the genetic material from the received cell samples. Next, the target genes are copied several million times. After this reproduction, a specific colouring technique makes it possible to identify which gene variants the test person is carrying. In just a couple of weeks the client receives a 'genetic profile' in the mail.

If it were up to Sciona the screening procedure at the high cost of 120 pounds sterling (175 Euros) would soon be offered in shops in the United States and continental Europe as well. Research director Gill-Garrison wants expansion. On the Internet, an international market has already established itself – and is already almost out of control. Alongside British and American suppliers, two companies, which sell genetic analyses freely over the Internet, have started operating across German-speaking regions. Physicians are excluded from this kind of testing business; according to professional law they are not allowed to advertise predictive tests. Paradoxically, this does not apply to the medical laity – thus an academically qualified engineer runs the Internet firm Gentest24 from Berlin. After receipt of a payment of between 500 and 1,600 Euros and a saliva sample, the enterprise gets a Berlin DNA laboratory to examine a number of genetic characteristics. The gene check allegedly reveals one's risk of developing Alzheimer's, breast cancer, cancer of the large intestine, osteoporosis, blood clotting problems and various metabolic diseases. Or, if you prefer, the Centre for Individual Diagnostic with its headquarters in Frankfurt-upon-Main can, it claims, determine genetic dispositions for cardiac infarct, obesity, addictive behaviour, menopausal problems and high blood pressure. The gene diagnostic for an 'anti-ageing-risk-profile' costs 653.61 Euros. Cunningly, the impression is created that gene tests are a prophylactic measure, just like abstaining from smoking: 'Only those who know their risks, can take preventive measures.'[1]

The US company Neuromark Diagnostics is currently searching for genes which are allegedly related to drug addiction, depression, compulsive eating habits, anxiety disorders and hyperactivity. All in all, it plans to come up with a set of between twenty and fifty key genes that could be used to predict human behaviour. Such a biotech crystal ball would be a sensation – and would of course be high-tech quackery. The reason: human behaviour is much too multifaceted to be foretold by gene-chip.

The service provided by the firm Sciona is similarly dubious. It is based on the fact that the genetic make-up of every human being is unique. Approximately one in every thousand pairs of bases differs from one person to the next, which generates at least 3 million deviations considering the total 3 billion building components.

This genetic diversity is a beneficial heritage of evolution, since it safeguards Homo sapiens' chances of survival – for example, when fighting menacing disease-causing agents. In the human genotype, many such variations lie dormant; biologists call them polymorphisms. They have the potential to affect the most diverse processes in the body. One polymorphism has, for example, the effect of making some people digest asparagus in a very peculiar way. It is possible to detect this after a meal oneself, as the affected person's urine smells unusually strong.

Anyway, once the 'gene profile' of a client has been established, Sciona employees cobble together a personalised report from fabricated diagnoses. It gives specific advice on nutrition in the light of the conducted gene analysis. At closer inspection, however, this turns out to be scientifically dressed-up nonsense. 'You & Your Genes' examines nine genes that play a role in metabolising nutrition. However, since six out of the nine genes have to do with the body's own detoxification, a certain variation in this area will most probably be found in most ᵃˢ, ᵃˢ ᵖᵘʳᵉˡʸ ˢᵗᵃᵗⁱˢᵗⁱᶜᵃˡ ʳᵉᵃˢᵒⁿˢ. Tᵒ ᵗᵒⁿᵉ ᵈᵒʷⁿ Sᶜⁱᵒⁿᵃ ᵃᵈᵛⁱˢᵉ ᵒⁿ ᶜˡᵃⁱᵐ-ing on such occasions, for instance, that key enzymes were working 'at speeds that are possibly not optimal for flushing out toxins from your body'. The woolly statements culminate in advice that applies to practically everyone. Abstain from eating charred meat and consume a lot of vegetables.

Other Sciona hints are equally banal. One is advised to take vitamin tablets and plenty of fruit. Cigarettes should be avoided and alcohol consumed in moderation. Sciona researcher Gill-Garrison admits that her expensive advice was not exactly original. 'There is surely no lack of good advice', she says, 'but our advice is probably more easily followed, because it is based on a completely personalised test. For the first time, we are telling people individually what's good for them based on their genes.'

It is precisely this claim, however, that is without any foundation. Even when the Sciona analysis shows that one gene is only partially functioning, this gives no concrete indication about whether general well-being will be affected. 'The alleged health consequences of the examined polymorphisms are largely unproven', criticises geneticist Peter Propping from the University of Bonn. Sciona relies on the ana-lyses of nine genes – whereas all in all, hundreds of different gene sequences play a role in digesting foods and metabolising them. How this complex interaction takes place is something that has still to be researched. 'We don't know yet exactly how genes and nutrition are correlated', says British scientist Roland Wolf from the University of Dundee. This is further compounded by the huge influence that the environment has on health.

It makes even less sense for Sciona to be testing the gene for 'aldehyde dehydrogenase', of which many Asians have an almost ineffective variant, for anyone who carries the defective enzyme will experience its bodily consequences early enough. Very small amounts of alcohol may trigger the concentration of a damaging by-product in the body – skin reddening, muzziness and heart racing are all symp-toms of this poisoning.

In the spring of 2002, a delegation from the British Human Genetics Commission inspected the newly consecrated Sciona laboratories and made the following comment: 'We are unaware of any sound scientific studies that have demonstrated that changing diet because of one's genetic make-up can alter health outcomes.'[2]

German experts are warning people against getting screened. 'This is all nonsense and doesn't say anything', pronounces, for instance, German geneticist Peter Propping. 'It is devastating, when such gene tests are offered on the free market.' Body Shop managers soon adopted this opinion: they removed the gene test from their product range after just a few months.

'You & Your Genes' gives one cause for thought in another regard. Each one of the allegedly inferior gene variants can be found in 20 to 40 per cent of the population. Consequently testers find five to six variants in most people. Statistically therefore, almost no one carries a perfect genetic make-up – according to the definition implied by Sciona. Hence, the test declares the vast majority of people genetically anomalous.

However, to date, these gene tests have not prevented a single disease. By contrast, they achieve quite the opposite effect: an expansion of the disease zone. For in the course of genetic scrutiny, trouble-free people are declared patients en masse.

'Our society is in the process of geneticisation', states Dutch philosopher Henk ten Have.

> As one aspect of the more comprehensive process of medicalisation, this process entails the redefinition of the individual in terms of the DNA code, a new language which describes and interprets human life and human behaviour according to a genetic vocabulary of codes, traits, drafts, dispositions and genetic make-up, as well as a genetic concept of disease, health and the human body.[3]

Fate by genetic referendum

Only in the case of some diseases can gene tests provide clarification. Approximately 280 diseases can now be diagnosed with gene testing, and this number will increase rapidly.[4] Looking at genes allows reliable prognoses for many hereditary diseases, namely for those conditions that are caused by a specific gene defect. The seemingly miniscule flaw can lead to the most severe symptoms and even death. In the case of these so-called monogenic diseases, gene tests can clearly determine who is ill and who is healthy. Therefore, not only can the future risks of an individual be predicted, but also interventions according to disease risks of the next generation can be made through pre-birth examinations and selective abortions. The number of monogenic diseases is estimated to be nearly 5,000. Thankfully, these are not common. Hamburg medical sociologists Günter Feuerstein and Regine Kollek put the figure at 'only 2 to 3 per cent of the total disease load'.[5]

As researchers explore the human genome, they simultaneously expand genetic diagnosis to diseases that are only partially genetically conditioned. Among them are, for example, cancer and cardiovascular diseases. In these common conditions, a puzzling profusion of genes plays a role alongside environmental influences – they are polygenic. Since 1982, for instance, more than twenty genes that are important for the transportation of fat through the blood have been discovered. If the interaction of these genes were out of kilter, this could promote the pathological hardening of blood vessel walls. The picture seems to be even more complex in the case of tumorous conditions. Researchers have already discovered more than sixty so-called proto-oncogenes. If these mutate, they can transform a healthy cell into a malignant cancerous one.

In the case of other polygenic diseases such as diabetes, Alzheimer's or thrombosis, researchers have also recently detected a multitude of genes of which little, if anything at all, is understood. The genetic part of common diseases occurs in patterns that have wide variation across the population's genetic pool and which, in any case, have only a moderate influence on the risk factor of any given disease.[6] Nevertheless, in the future researchers hope to be able to give reliable prognoses about disease risks based on these genetic patterns – although they would have to achieve the enormous feat of adequately accounting for the combined effects of environmental factors.

At the present, however, gene tests do not reveal when exactly a polygenic disease will break out and how it will develop – even though private gene interpreters like the companies Sciona and Gentest24 seem to be suggesting something to the contrary. But because polygenic variants are so widespread, it is likely to become big business. Companies like Roche and Novartis cooperate with small biotech firms that are developing new types of tests.[7]

The gene inspection provides – if anything – purely statistical statements about risks. One is simply playing with probabilities. Tricky, given, on the one hand, the extent to which the average person who tested 'positive' is likely to understand statistics. Further, it may have the effect of scare mongering. An explicit example in the United States is the widespread, commercial gene test for hereditary cancer of the breast and the ovaries. American producer Myriad Genetic Laboratories approaches women directly in its advertisements. 'Does breast or ovarian cancer run in your family? You can reduce the risk. We can help.'

It is true that the expensive gene test – it costs around 2,500 Euros – can determine whether a woman carries one of the cancer genes BRCA1 or BRCA2. What it cannot do, though, is to predict whether the disease will actually develop. Women who test positive then have to decide whether they want to have their ovaries removed or to have their breasts amputated as a prophylactic measure. A number of American and German women have undergone surgery, even though it appears that 40 to 50 per cent of carriers do not develop breast cancer and 80 per cent do not get ovarian cancer.

Even in the case of well-researched hereditary diseases, the genes may be misguiding. In the most common hereditary disease in Central Europe, cystic fibrosis, 3 to 5 per cent of carriers of homozygous characteristics do not become ill.

The sequencing of the human genome will bring thousands of genetic variants to light, tempting doctors to describe them as anomalous, undesirable and pathological traits – and so the stage is once more being set for disease mongering opportunism to make its entrance.

British scientists David Melzer and Ron Zimmern warn against sorting people into pigeonholes of 'healthy' or 'ill', based on their genetic characteristics. 'On a fundamental level, genetic science is forcing a re-examination of the concept of normality itself, by showing that everyone's genome is different and that we are all in some sense "abnormal".'[8]

Even though the genetic profile seems to suggest something different – only conditions that diminish or jeopardise a patient's well-being should be considered diseases. One example of a bodily phenomenon, which can be clearly diagnosed, yet is harmless to one's health, is the so-called Gilbert's syndrome. Affected persons have an elevated level of liver enzymes when they are exposed to stress. Many more such variants, which might be scientifically interesting yet do not have any detrimental health consequences, are hidden in the human genome.

Canadian physician Larissa Temple also warns, in *Science* magazine, of labelling trouble-free people as patients solely on the basis of their genetic profile: 'Until a mutation is shown to demonstrate a defined risk of developing adverse consequences, individuals carrying that mutation should not be considered diseased.' In the genetic make-up of humans, researchers will find myriads of slight genetic variations. To define their harmful consequences and adequately determine their risks is a mammoth, perhaps impossible task.[9]

Most of nature's whims – earlobes attached to the head to give the notable example mentioned earlier – are evenly scattered among populations and often do not stand out at all. If they lead to symptoms, their severity, in turn, may vary from one person to another – genes do not draw any sharp dividing lines. In order to differentiate between 'diseased' and 'healthy' in this commission established by nature, physicians make do with arbitrary criteria that are subject to fashion – as is so often the case in medicine. 'Over time, the tendency has been to expand diagnostic and treatment boundaries', observe researchers David Melzer and Ron Zimmern from Cambridge, England. Consequently, they say, people with milder pathological manifestations and lower risk levels have increasingly been included in the 'disease' category.

Modern medicine reinforces this tendency, Melzer and Zimmern warn. Tests for genetic traits (markers) that 'may not result in symptoms for half a century or more could be new examples of a process of premature medicalisation, of attaching the "disease" label before it has been established that prevention or treatment is clearly beneficial'.[10]

This way, the genome becomes a medical risk factor, and diagnosis transgresses the boundaries more than ever. A healthy person is one whose genetic make-up has not, or has not *yet*, been examined thoroughly enough.

Genetic test results, even though scientifically they might say little or nothing about a person's future state of health, can be used deliberately to depict people as anomalous or diseased. The obvious consequence is that anyone who carries a supposed flaw runs the risk of being unfairly treated by insurers and employers.

In Germany private health and life insurers have voluntarily declared that they will not demand gene tests or ask to look at existing results, until the year 2006 at the earliest. However, this applies only to insurance amounts up to 250,000 Euros. If higher amounts are involved existing results have to be presented.

Genes and fallacies

A glance at the USA demonstrates the need to defuse this potential time bomb. At least six American companies are already screening applicants to determine whether they are particularly sensitive to certain toxic substances that they might come into contact with during their work. Those that are deemed so are not offered employment. People with a gene for the so-called sickle-cell anaemia were also refused certain jobs in the United States, even though the affected persons were only carriers of the trait and otherwise in good health. In this condition, if both versions of the gene are mutated, red blood cells in affected people's bodies become lumpy and crescent shaped when a lack of oxygen occurs. In the 1970s, the US Air Force restricted even the admission of symptom-free carriers into its academy; commercial airlines employed them only as ground staff, but not as cabin crew or pilots. The genetic discrimination mainly hit black US citizens since black people carry this gene variant more often. After fierce protests, the restrictions were lifted.[11]

In the years to come, a number of new variants that could lead to similar fallacies and discriminations will undoubtedly be discovered in the human genetic make-up. But when people hear about supposed flaws in their genome, it might cause them anxiety or even deprive them of their courage to go on living. 'A test result which names a more or less certain statistical risk seems like a mortgage that burdens the life of a healthy person', argue experts Günter Feuerstein and Regine Kollek from Hamburg. As the number of genetic diagnoses grows, the number of people who do not understand the complex test result and who are left alone with their fears grows too. 'The increasing awareness that identifiable genetic factors participate in the development of almost every disease will not remain without social consequences', warns geneticist Jörg Schmidtke from the Medical School in Hanover, Germany. The 'flaw in the genetic make-up' would also become a 'flaw of the persons themselves'.

We all know that one might suddenly develop a severe disease – a disease that might even turn out to be fatal. But this usually suppressed possibility is turned into an acute and inescapable threat by a positive gene test – no matter how speculative it might be. New categories of patients emerge: 'the healthy ill' and 'the not yet ill'.

In the near future, medical care for this new patient group will become a staple part of the health system, particularly since gene tests will be applied more and more extensively. For the pharmaceutical industry, this opens up a huge market. The industry's target is the development of medicaments for people who do not have any symptoms, but carry an anomalous gene pattern. In the past the 'apple a day' was enough to keep the doctor away; nowadays, for those supposedly predisposed to cardiac infarct, 'an aspirin a day' could be recommended to thin the blood; others, whom biology has burdened with Alzheimer's could, similarly, be administered memory pills as a purely prophylactic measure, and so on, and so on. Preventive medicine used to have the goal of keeping people away from the health system – in the age of genetic diagnosis people are guided towards it.

The relatively common hemochromatosis provides an example of how genome research is already encouraging medicalisation. Textbooks tell us the hereditary disease occurs in one out of every 400 people. The affected persons are trouble free, but accumulate a surplus of iron in their bodies, which may lead to conditions in later life such as liver cirrhosis, diabetes and cardiac insufficiency. The surplus iron and subsequent damage could be avoided by regular blood transfusions – if only those people were aware early enough of their hereditary disease. In the course of an unprecedented mass screening, the health insurance institution Kaufmännische Krankenkasse in Hanover, Germany, examined 6,000 insured persons to detect potential hemochromatosis. But it turned out that less than 1 per cent of people who carry the respective mutated gene subsequently become ill. Thus gene tests 'for hemochromatosis identify a genetic risk rather than the disease itself', argues Wylie Burke from the University of Washington in Seattle. The dilemma is whether to turn ninety-nine people into healthy sufferers in order to prevent one from becoming sick.[12]

Medical sociologist Feuerstein from Hamburg, who researches the effects of gene checks on health insurance, warns about huge follow-up costs: 'In the future, trouble-free people will be turned *en masse* into patients. It would be financial madness if people were to be treated from their youth onwards with medicaments and therapies.' If this happened, gene tests could be the financial ruin of public health insurance schemes.

Just being healthy is not enough

The prevention of hereditary conditions and eradication of disease-causing genes has had a place in science since 1883. At that time, an Englishman by the name of Francis Galton, cousin of the natural scientist Charles Darwin, founded eugenics and established its first institute, the Galton Laboratory in London. The scholar considered Britons insufficiently equipped both mentally and physically to rule their vast empire. Through use of eugenics (from Greek 'wellborn'), he wanted to augment desirable hereditary dispositions in the population.

At the beginning of the twentieth century eugenics was a popular theory that found quite a variety of applications – particularly when eradicating undesirable hereditary dispositions was involved. In Norway and Sweden, mentally ill people, criminals and homosexuals were sterilised. Eugenics gave Germans the grounds for discrimination and genocide. On 18 August 1939, an obligation to notify the authorities of births of deformed babies was enacted. In the long term, Nazi Germany was to be 'cleansed' of disabled people. In the USA, at least 60,000 men and women were compulsorily sterilised up until the 1970s because of alleged hereditary diseases. In December 2002, this led the governor of Oregon to make a public apology for the fact that more than 2,600 people in his state were sterilised against their will.

The theory of hereditary health has been given a new lease of life by modern biology. English geneticists Gordon Ferns and David Galton write that eugenics was nowadays to be defined as 'the use of science applied to the qualitative and quantitative improvement of the human genome'.[13] Based on the knowledge of presumed and real disease genes currently being located in the thickets of genomes, both these goals of eugenics may be pursued.

Supposed 'bad' hereditary dispositions are eliminated. Based on their individual gene endowment, certain people find themselves in the biological lower classes. For them, it is much more difficult to find work, and they are rarely promoted. It is also difficult for them to get credit, health insurance and life insurance – all factors that reduce the reproduction prospects of affected people.

Supposed 'good' hereditary dispositions are increased. Artificially produced embryos are genetically screened, and only the desired ones implanted in the womb. The technique (pre-implantation diagnostics) has been used by physicians and parents on an estimated 1,000 children. Most of these cases so far have been solely for the prevention of the most serious hereditary conditions. But the search for gene patterns of polygenic conditions and anomalies continues.

In Chicago, a 30-year-old woman, herself a geneticist, got her artificially fertilised embryos tested for a mutation that can lead to the early onset of Alzheimer's disease. Four of the embryos that did not show any mutation were implanted in the woman, and one of them grew into a child. Without the screening, the baby would have had a fifty-fifty risk of growing up with the prospect of being incurably ill by the age of 40. Instead, the woman gave birth to a healthy girl.[14]

In rare cases, even a healthy genome is not enough to guarantee the implantation of an embryo – for instance, in the case of a genetically predetermined baby that is supposed to function as an organ donor. The first child of this kind was named Adam Nash. The boy was born into the world in the autumn of 2002 as a saviour baby. Only seconds after his birth in an American clinic, physicians took blood from his umbilical cord and later rinsed cells from it into the body of his sister. For anaemic Molly, at that time 6, her brother's donation was the ultimate in medicine – it had no side effects.

The little saviour was not heaven-sent, but selected by a geneticist. Adam was reproduced in vitro together with around a dozen other embryos. In the laboratory dish, physicians subjected the embryos to a genetic test. Adam passed it. Because his tissue characteristics were best suited to match his sister's, his mother carried and gave birth only to him – as a son and as a donor.

'We've crossed the line that we really never had crossed before', stated bio-ethicist Jeffrey Kahn from the University of Minnesota at the time, 'selecting based on characteristics that are not the best for the child being born, but for somebody else.' The beginning of a new era? Manfred Stauber from the Women's Clinic at the University of Munich fears so. His concern is that the production of 'children who are as suitable as possible, might become a principle of practice'.[15]

Adam, the bouncing baby boy born in the US state of Colorado, is the harbinger of an unknown medicine. His genes are 'good' through use of eugenics. Good for him and at the same time beneficial for another person. Adam is more than just healthy.

11 Healthy beyond belief

> If you carry on like this, no one will want to be sick any more.
>
> Molière

The disease trade promises us a destiny similar to that of the inhabitants of Saint Maurice, the mountain village where Dr Knock practised. In the end, only as many citizens are allowed to remain healthy as are needed to care for the army of ailing in the newly converted infirmary. Germany is on its way to being transformed into this hospital. Already, at any one time, there are more than half a million German citizens in hospital, while almost 15 million – just about one-fifth of the population – are being treated as inpatients in hospitals every year. If this transformation progresses unchecked, in the near future every German will either work for the health system or be treated by it – or both.

The advance of medicine into the personal and social realms of life has led to its unprecedented expansion. Never before, in the societies of western industrial nations, has it been as powerful as it is nowadays. The triumph of medicine has brought about three paradoxical consequences. First, the cost of the health system is increasing exponentially – with no equivalent gain in health. Second, physicians are becoming disillusioned – the number of medical doctors who regret their choice of profession has risen dramatically. Third, people are not in any better health – if anything, they are feeling sicker and sicker.

Paradox 1: a high price to pay for no benefit

The extensive medicalisation of our lives contributes directly to the fact that health systems are no longer financially feasible. Expenditure on statutory health insurance climbs year after year to new record heights: from 97.6 billion Euros in 1991 to 145 billion Euros in 2003. In Germany alone, 4.1 million people are earning a living in the health system. This amounts to living off other people's ill health

If the disease in our society were a 'finite' entity, competition in the medical professions would lead to a favourable and benevolent medicine, speculated the late American expert Lynn Payer. 'But since disease is such a fluid and political concept, the providers can essentially create their own demand by broadening the definitions of disease [in such a way as to include the greatest number of people, and by spinning out new diseases].'[1] The currently observable plundering of health systems is the consequence.

But when healthy people take away really ill people's right to benefit from the resources, the integrity of the health insurance system is called into question. The prescription of hormones to women who are regarded as diseased solely because they are menopausal costs German public health insurers around 500 million Euros every year. Truly exorbitant are the statins, those supposed miracle pills, which seem to lower the risk of cardiovascular diseases. The European Society of Cardiologists advocates prescribing the remedy widely. But if their heart protection programme were implemented, at their current market price the necessary statins would cost 19 billion Euros yearly, that is two-thirds of the German budget for medicaments (32.4 billion Euros in 2000).[2] The logic of our health system, however, is based on the fact that the financial resources should benefit the 20 per cent of the population who are ill – and not the remaining 80 per cent of the perhaps 'healthy ill' as well. Funding frittered away on unnecessary treatments could be better invested elsewhere, for example, for the treatment of serious diseases or for improving working conditions in hospitals. Treating affluent citizens of the lifestyle society seems shameful if one considers how many lives could be saved in developing countries with this money, through hygiene measures, access to clean water and vaccinations.

Paradox 2: disillusioned doctors

Being a doctor is no longer as rewarding as it used to be. Nowadays, general practitioners are almost happy to see a patient with a real disease: someone they can actually help from time to time. At least every other person attending a consultation complains about a disease that is not detectable. The healthy people persuaded into surgeries by worries spread by disease mongers increase doctors' workload and their frustration. While the health industry creates an increased demand for medicine, doctors are left to manage the shortfall since their budget does not rise. Moreover, medicalisation leads to society simply offloading the unpleasant concomitants of life, such as old age and pain, onto the family doctor. Often, doctors are regarded as the cause for medicalisation, but they are to a large extent its victims.

Constantin Rössner, general practitioner in Bad Neuenahr, Germany, has had enough. When he read an article in a journal for doctors stating that excess weight – pardon, adiposity – should be recognised as a disease, he finally blew his top. One should rather 'try a new definition of health for a change, and differentiate it from the treatment of diseases', Rössner wrote in a reader's letter.

> Instead, medicine spins out ever new and prohibitive diseases which are, in the end, social problems ('Adiposity is still not regarded as a disease in these parts' – what a shame!). If we waved goodbye to our omnipotent pomposity and exercised some modesty instead, then many problems would simply vanish overnight. Let's stick with the ancient Egyptians. For them, only what they were able to treat was a disease.[3]

Paradox 3: worrying ourselves sick

This is the biggest paradox of modern medicine. The richer a country is and the more money a society pumps into its health system, the higher the probability that its society's members feel ill. In many cases, early diagnoses and prevention do not prolong life – instead they increase the number of unhappy years. Amartya Sen, Nobel Prize winner for economics, has investigated and compared how people in two states of India judge their well-being. In the rich state of Kerala, there are only a few illiterate people, and on average every inhabitant goes once a year to the doctor. Life expectancy is, at 74 years, considerably high. Strangely, however, the inhabitants assess their health as being rather poor.

In the poorer state of Bihar, on the other hand, statistically citizens hardly ever reach the age of 60 and only one out of five Biharians ever seeks medical treatment – in spite of this, an extremely low percentage of people in Bihar claim to feel ill. The preoccupation with aches and pains is linked with a higher level of education, suspects Amartya Sen. In contrast to their rich contemporaries, the state of people in poorer regions was less troubled by 'the awareness of treatable conditions to be distinguished from "natural" states of being'.[4]

In a world where the truth lies in perception, one is hence better off with less medicine.

Made ill through medicine

Superfluous therapies turn many healthy people into patients for good. In Germany, every year 40,000 accusations of professional errors are made, of which almost 12,000 are proven to be real treatment errors. Very often medicaments become a danger. At German chemists, there are 50,000 ready-made drugs on offer, although the index of indispensable medicaments published by the World Health Organisation contains only 325 active agents.[5] Each year, 20,000 people in Germany die as a result of medications; their side effects are the cause of 2 to 3 per cent of all hospitalisations, which leads to costs amounting to around 500 million Euros. An American analysis reveals that undesirable effects of drugs are, in medically high-tech industrial nations, the fourth most common cause of death after coronary heart diseases, tumorous diseases and strokes, but before pneumonia, diabetes and accidents.[6]

It is yet unknown to what extent disease mongering is contributing to the excess pill popping. However, it is rather the norm than the exception that people take several drugs together. 'It seems hard to believe', says a medical magazine, 'but some patients are in fact treated with 60 or more substances at the same time.'[7] Approximately 22 per cent of all side effects can be attributed to taking too many drugs indiscriminately.

Just plain healthy just isn't good enough

The medicalisation of our existence makes people feel discontent with their bodies – hence, a cosmetic medicine emerges. It does not cure the ill, it improves the healthy. Thus, some American managers are already requesting prophylactic bypass surgery. In neurotechnology (technology affecting brain patterns) a multitude of substances is emerging which could misleadingly be applied to serve self-optimisation. The psycho-pharmaceutical Prozac and its numerous successors, taken by healthy people as happy pills, are only the beginning. Pharmaceutical companies scour the human psyche for states to be perfected. Remedies for shyness, forgetfulness, sleepiness and stress are being tested in clinical studies or soon will be.

The trend towards making the normal treatable can be seen, for instance, in short or slow-growing children. Their parents and paediatricians find themselves under pressure to treat them with growth hormones. The affected children are assumed to be socially and psychologically disadvantaged, which, however, cannot be proven scientifically.[8]

The research on 'mild cognitive impairment' – the occasional mental vagueness which can occur naturally in older age – is another example of how normal behaviour is being cured. Companies such as Californian Cortex Pharmaceuticals and Targacept in the US state of North Carolina are currently researching a substance that is supposed to intervene in the chemical processes of the brain and thereby keep the memory young.[9]

In their search for the clever pill, scientists from Stanford University, California have perhaps already made a find. The remedy Aricept, which is normally administered only to Alzheimer's patients, was given to nine healthy airplane pilots for thirty days. The anti-dementia medication alters the brain's chemistry by blocking the enzyme acetylcholinesterase. This effect could also be shown in the case of the pilots. After taking the medication, the pilots performed better in flight simulator tests than they had in their previous attempts. In direct comparison with nine other pilots who did not take pills, the pilots who took Aricept also appeared superior. Will future chess champions and Nobel Prize winners also optimise their mental powers by taking such 'cogniceuticals'?

The answer will probably be yes. There is no lack of people who are discontent with their god-given faculties and physique and want to perfect themselves with surgery and pharmaceuticals. Even when physical anomalies are imaginary, 'affected' people experience them as real. In most cases, the supposed flaw is of the face, breasts or genitals. Medics talk about a 'shame-disease'.

Dr Ruthild Linse, head of the Dermatology Clinic at the Helios Hospital Erfurt, says, 'Things, such as old age, obesity, being unfit and having inadequate body hair, are more likely to trigger feelings of shame than being naked'. In her surgery, she has observed a 'sharp increase in patients with dysmorphic body disorders', which she attributes to marketing strategies in the cosmetic and pharmaceutical industries. Linse and two of her colleagues write in the journal *Deutsches Ärzteblatt*:

> Additional thematicalisation of dermatological cosmetology in the media (lifestyle magazines, private TV stations and Internet), as

well as licensing of fashion dependent lifestyle medicaments for hair growth, potency and weight reduction have resulted in a swift and strong parallel increase in patient consultations with cosmetic questions, as well as in a rapidly increasing demand for treatment.

In the physicians' opinion, a high proportion of the advice-seekers – up to 23 per cent – were, in reality, psychologically disturbed.

Joie de vivre or life of fear

In their quest for beauty, people demand lifestyle medicaments or otherwise fall into the clutches of cosmetic surgery, but this does not always solve their problem. Affected persons often pay high prices for their 'artificial' noses, ears, breasts or hips – and are still not content with their new body parts. The latest craze of beauty addicts is the bacterial toxin botulinum, which temporarily affects human nerve cells, and can be used for facial anti-wrinkle injections and per-spiration reduction – for a while. Even some people who sweat normally insist on botulinum toxin (Botox) therapy. The derma-tologists from Erfurt have suggested a new clinical picture, which they claim to have diagnosed in around one-fifth of their patients: 'Botulinophilia'.[10]

This and other so-called dysmorphic body disorders are regarded as a sub-form of hypochondria. Between 1 and 3 per cent of Germans suffer from this pathological fear of disease – so rough estimates report. That this condition is being expanded to include a slightly less pronounced variant sounds strangely familiar. Psychologists Gaby Bleichhardt and Wolfgang Hiller from the University of Mainz surveyed the health of 2,000 Germans and claim to have made a strike. Accordingly, 7 per cent of the population are suffering from 'pronounced disease fears'. That progressing medicalisation deepens, expands and finally elevates these worries to the status of treatment-requiring symptoms, seems to foster a state of affairs in which any sense of *joie de vivre* is eroded away, laying bare in its place the raw fear of life.

This obsession with health has already been named in the English language: healthism. According to English physician James Le Fanu, it is 'a medically inspired obsession with trivial or non-existent threats to health whose assertions would in the past, quite rightly, have been dismissed as quackery'.[11]

The phenomenon of healthism places the causes of all problems as well as their solutions firmly with the individual. By transfiguring health into an ideal, into a comprehensive metaphor for quality of life, healthism reinforces the tendency to depict the human struggle to achieve the best state of health possible, as a private and personal matter. In other words, the blame for problems and diseases is attached to the individual – leaving politics and society to slink out of sight, shirking their responsibility.

The alleged epidemic of hyperactive children is just one example. If there were a million – or even just a hundred thousand – primary pupils lacking in concentration to the point of behavioural disorder, is it really conceivable that the cause for this mass phenomenon could lie solely with each child? The idea of drugging these children into submission rather than looking for the causes of their behaviour in the environment – in the parental home and to a lesser degree in kindergartens and schools – and attempting changes there instead is wholly unacceptable. Another example is the army of supposed patients with no detectable disease. The question as to whether the causes for their ailing can in fact be attributed to the individuals themselves, must be raised here too. Are their defence mechanisms against stress too weak – or have environmental stress factors simply become too overwhelming for many people?

Why the poor die younger

It is a well-known fact that the environment has a decisive influence on the state of a person's health. 'Poor in the pocket, ill at heart', wrote Goethe and his words still ring true nowadays. In the industrialised countries, health chances decrease in proportion with income. 'Compared with managers, simple workers have three times the risk of suffering cardiac infarct', says Johannes Siegrist, medical sociologist at the University of Düsseldorf. The German cardiovascular disease prevention study involving 10,000 people showed that in the lower fifth of the population cardiovascular diseases occur twice as often as in the upper fifth. Science calls this a 'social gradient'; it divides society into a healthy upper class and sickly middle to lower classes. Epidemiologists noticed the gradient also with relation to asthma, diabetes, obesity, depression and slipped discs.[12]

Unhealthy lifestyles, however, account for only half of the social gradient in cardiovascular diseases, says Johannes Siegrist. This was proven by many studies that compared groups at risk. That rich smokers live longer than poor smokers is one of the results.

But how can the remaining 50 per cent of the social gradient be explained? Why do people from the lower sections suffer from high blood pressure, cardiac infarct, stroke or angina pectoris more often when life circumstances are similarly healthy or unhealthy, when medical care is to a large extent the same for everybody and when genetic factors do not play a role either?

The social gradient is evidently linked to biochemical processes, for instance the secretion of stress hormones. Researchers believe they have proven in a number of studies that the body reacts with biochemical responses to financial need and social strain. One of the most reliable studies comes from Sweden. When factory workers there lost their jobs, they increasingly produced cholesterol, fibrinogen and stress hormones – physiological alterations that favour the pathological constriction of blood vessels.

Not unemployment and poverty alone, but 'the correlation between performance and reward' was responsible for the biochemical changes, says Siegrist. 'Anyone who, without a chance of professional advancement, has to do heavy work for years while also fearing redundancy, seems to be at risk.' In his view, prevailing expert medical opinion restricts itself too much to classical risk factors. Siegrist's conclusion: 'Diseases can only be prevented, if one comprehends their social dimensions.'[13]

Unfortunately, this concept finds no place in the disease mongers' philosophy. They stand diametrically opposed to such views, holding the individual responsible for his or her state of health. The affected persons are thereby stigmatised, which can be shown again in the example of hyperactive children. Their behaviour is no longer tolerated, because it annoys and seems too different from the norm. The willingness to accept differing ways of life is diminishing. To the same extent, the number of psychiatric diagnoses is rising. Society has an increasingly low tolerance for unusual behaviour. These are bad times for oddballs and eccentrics.

In the near future as our knowledge of genetics increases, so stigmatising because of diseases will also increase tremendously. Every human probably carries three to five mutations for a recessive hereditary condition (disease breaks out only when both genes, from the mother's and the father's side, are mutated). Hence, it is very likely that a great number of genes, triggering or favouring diseases in later life, will be discovered in the near future; among them possibly even the hypothesised 'disease genes' related to socially undesirable behaviour. This will have an unprecedented impact on our image of health, according to Australian ethicists Jacinta Kerin and Julian

Savulescu: 'In a sense, genetics will enable us to see that we are all "diseased" in some ways.'[14]

Perhaps the most serious misdeed of disease mongering lies in the way it nourishes the idea that health can be bought like goods in a store. Processes and difficulties in life, such as birth, sexuality, ageing, frustration, tiredness, loneliness and ugliness, are being medicalised more and more. Medicine cannot solve these problems. The effect it does have, however, is to undermine the human ability to accept pain, illness and even death.

Winding up in hospital

'Life in hospital is bitter', observed physician and poet Gottfried Benn, 'one dies there, without vine leaves in one's hair.' Nowadays, every second German citizen passes away in hospital; most of them die of what was formerly called old age. 'In ambulances with blue lights flashing, very old, dying people are brought in . . . Totally dreadful', says physician Johannes Bolte from the General Hospital Altona in Hamburg. Quickly, the diagnostic machine is running at full speed. Physicians take blood and urine from the elderly persons and push them swiftly, before it's too late, into the tube-shaped computer tomograph – in hospital no one is allowed to expect a beautiful death.[15]

Medical critic Ivan Illich wrote:

> Consciously lived frailty, individuality and socialization of the human being make experiences of pain, illness and death an essential part of human life. The ability to cope with these three things autonomously is the basis of human health. If human beings become dependent on the bureaucratic administration of their intimate realm, they renounce their autonomy. In truth, the miracle of medicine is a devilish illusion. It consists in getting, not only individuals, but whole sections of the population to survive on an inhumanly low level of personal health.[16]

In the late 1970s, Illich's analysis was revolutionary – now sections of the medical establishment recognise truth in what he had to say. In its hubris, medicine is threatening the health of human beings. 'The cost of trying to defeat death, pain and sickness is unlimited, and beyond a certain point every penny spent may make the problem worse, eroding still further the human capacity to cope with reality.'[17]

Even though the boundaries of medical science are expanding further and further, it is time to draw the line; it is time for a comprehensive 'demedicalisation'. It would be unrealistic, though, to expect the health industry to voluntarily commit itself to such a process. The industry seems oblivious. 'The pharmaceutical market is currently concerned less with meeting health needs and more with the growth requirements of the industry', pronounces London researcher David Gilbert, 'The goals of healthcare policy are in danger of becoming subsidiary to those of the pharmaceutical industry.'[18] No reform or improvement is to be expected from Dr Knock's successors then. Protected by the freedom of therapy, physicians are becoming blasé about the invention of diseases and so will continue in the same way they have gone on.

Nevertheless, there are a few therapies that can help deal with the syndrome of disease mongering. Here are five suggestions:

1 The British Nuffield Council in Bioethics recommends charging a separate agency with monitoring and controlling 'the deliberate medicalising of normal populations'.[19] In Germany too, the establishment of an independent, publicly funded monitoring body is overdue: a 'product test foundation' for diseases. The foundation, whose members would also include medical laity, would reveal fabricated conditions, throw them out of the service catalogue and publish generally comprehensible dossiers on scientifically founded clinical pictures, syndromes and disorders, preferably on the Internet. This way, general practitioners, journalists and last but not least citizens would have access to independent information.

2 Information on diseases and therapies is often based on ill-informed, one-sided studies that typically involve only a few patients, that are restricted to short periods of time and that have been subjected to industry's influence. That companies are not required to provide data about the long-term benefits and the side effects of drugs is simply wrong. Many companies withhold funding for more thorough clinical studies, preferring instead to invest the money in marketing activities. Conceivably, such studies could be financed from an independent research pool, to which the industry would be formally obliged to make contributions.

3 As a matter of course, physicians should be encouraged to attend continuing education courses organised independently from the industry. Peter Schönhöfer, Professor of Clinical Pharmacology and co-publisher of the critical *arznei-telegramm*, calls upon his colleagues in the medical profession to exercise more scepticism:

Physicians are much too uncritical of the way the pharmaceutical industry advertises its new products. I think that the most urgent reform in medical studies should be to provide students with a thorough understanding of how to read between the lines of the industry's misinformation.[20]

4   The extent of the financial connections between pharmaceutical companies and physicians has become obscured to a degree that jeopardises the image and independence of medicine. It is time to make these ties transparent and subject to regulation. The medical profession itself is putting up particular resistance to the intimate relationship the industry is courting. Physician Arne Schäffler from Bavarian Kiefersfelden says, 'What we physicians want least of all is to be seen in the public eye as a corruptible, venal profession. But the seeds of this have already been sown.'[21] Medical doctor Schäffler has worked himself in a leading position at the marketing department of a pharmaceutical company and knows how the industry's manipulation works. Schäffler demands a 'Code of Conduct', which German doctors should impose on themselves through their self-government agencies. It should list which connections and financial contributions between industry and doctors ought to be allowed and which not, as well as give grounds for these judgements. As a general rule, all financial ties between companies and medical doctors should be brought out into the open, in scientific articles, expert judgements and press bulletins.

5   Good medicine knows its bounds and refuses to turn each and every sphere and phase of life into an object of medical intervention. Critical doctors are proposing a prescription against stalking healthy people with unnecessary therapies: so-called evidence-based medicine. When general practitioners, for instance, use preventive medicine or therapy, they should be obliged to provide conclusive, scientific proof that these measures will have some benefit. Introducing evidence-based medicine is, according to Heiner Raspe from the Institute for Social Medicine at the University Clinic Lübeck, imperative for the credibility of the art of healing. 'The contract between society and medicine is in need of a new foundation.'[22] Without the slightest effort, each medical doctor could work on restoring the trust between patient and doctor. All the doctor needs to do is to remember one medical virtue: to leave the healthy in peace.

Don't worry, be happy

This is not about trivialising real diseases. Anyone who is suffering from a disease consults the doctor – no questions asked. But everybody else should stand resolute in their determination not to be seduced by the trappings offered by the disease mongers. Back in 1840 therapist Bernhard Hirschel already knew: 'People far and wide want to believe in the possibility of a panacea to cure all disease or to believe in the power of those who claim to be able to do so.'[23]

Nowadays, many older, but increasingly also younger people allow themselves to be lured all too willingly by the booming medical-industrial complex. Visits to the doctor combat loneliness and boredom. The connection to the health industry represents a kind of socialisation, maintains physician Bernard Lown. It gives people 'comfort to have someone who listens attentively to their problems'.[24] In reality, even the particularly intelligent seem to abandon all reason when it comes to their health, which makes them especially susceptible to the persuasions of disease mongers. The remedy for this is a huge dose of calmness and composure. Happily, there are still medical doctors who do prescribe exactly this. Physicians Petr Skrabanek and James McCormick write:

> Since life itself is a universally fatal sexually transmitted disease, living it to the full demands a balance between reasonable and unreasonable risk. Because this balance is a matter of judgment, dogmatism has little place. Present-day preoccupations with health are largely unhealthy as the media constantly draw to our attention hazards to health. Many of these hazards are rare and our individual risk of being harmed extremely small; in this circumstance they should be ignored.[25]

Healthy . . . who me?

Less belief in physicians and more scepticism can help you to discover your own health. Diagnoses and diseases are not laws of nature; they are based on agreements made by interested parties. Anyone who is asked to attend a check-up and leaves with a diagnosis should keep this fact in mind and not hesitate to ask the doctor who exactly has determined that the diagnosed condition is in fact a disease: what knowledge in medical science proves that this condition will harm me? To what extent can medical measures improve my condition? If a hundred people are treated, how many of them will benefit? What scientific evidence is there to support the proposed therapy?

The Internet weakens physicians' power and increases patients' knowledge. Cancer patients, for example, have been using the Internet for quite some time now to collect information about their diseases and the optimal therapy. They exchange facts worth knowing, support and reassure each other in emails and confront their doctor with 'snips' from the Internet. Just like diseased people who want to become healthy, healthy people who refuse to be taken for a ride as patients, can also find valuable information on the Internet (see pages 152–53 for a list of relevant databases and search engines).

Equipped with knowledge about the natural life course, its stages and conditions, people would be in a much better position to make informed decisions when confronted with medicine's ever-new claims and instructions. It is true, however, that much information is still not easy to find. State involvement would therefore be desirable to support and subsidise, for instance, consumer protection agencies enabling them to be more informative and to raise public awareness specifically about diseases and the medicalisation of life.

But everyone already has the possibility of making up their own mind about their health and should trust their own judgements more. Everyone can choose whether or not to be admitted, weighed and measured, inspected, admonished, discussed, injected, X-rayed, poked, cupped, anointed, plastered, cut and stitched, genetically tested, treated by radiation, fed with pills, put on a diet and to have thermometers inserted à la Dr Knock.

Everyone has the choice to disregard, slight, snub and turn their backs on the disease mongers. At the end of the day, you are only sick if you have been diagnosed so.

Appendix
Twelve questions to diagnose invented diseases and dubious treatments

1 Is there a name for my illness?
2 Are there international guidelines describing diagnosis and treatment of this illness and if so, where can I read about them?
3 Is there a test that can clearly identify my illness?
4 In how many healthy persons does this test show a positive (pathological) result?
5 For people who tested positive, can repetition of the test result in a normal outcome? If so, for what percentage of people?
6 What is the proportion of false negative results? (How many people are not diagnosed by the test, but do actually have the disease?)
7 What are the potential consequences of this disease for me in one, two, ten years' time and in what percentage of people like me do these consequences actually occur after one, two, ten years?
8 In what percentage of people who *do not have* this disease can these complications occur anyway in one, two, ten years?
9 Is there an effective treatment for this disease?
10 In what percentage of people who are like me, and who *undergo* this treatment, do these complications *still occur* in one, two, ten years?
11 In what percentage of people who are like me, and who *do not undergo* the treatment, do these complications occur in one, two, ten years?
12 In what percentage of people who are like me, and who *undergo* the treatment, do complications *related to treatment* occur, which would not have occurred otherwise?

Source: Prof. Dr Peter Sawicki from DIeM Institute for Evidence-based Medicine in Cologne.

Notes

1 Limitless healing

1 Quoted from L. Payer, *Disease Mongers*, New York, 1992, and according to J. Romaine, *Knock ou le Triomphe de la Médecine*, Stuttgart, 1989.
2 *Der Spiegel* 47, 2002.
3 R. Moynihan and R. Smith, 'Too much medicine?', *British Medical Journal* 324, 2002, 859–60.
4 M. Burgmer, 'Das "Sisi"-Syndrom – eine neue Depression?', *Der Nervenarzt* 74, 2003. Online. Available: http://www.wedopress.de (accessed 22. 5. 2003).
5 *Herald Tribune*, 4. 1. 2003.
6 *Ärzte Zeitung*, 8. 4. 2002.
7 *Ärzte Zeitung*, 16. 12. 2002.
8 U. Streeck, 'Die generalisierte Heiterkeitsstörung', *Forum der Psychoanalyse* 16, 2000, 116–22; the contribution was supposed to be a satire, which many readers failed to notice.
9 R. Moynihan, 'Drug firms hype disease as sales ploy, industry chief claims', *British Medical Journal* 324, 2002, 867.
10 H. S. Füeßl, 'Neue Krankheiten braucht das Land!', *MMW-Fortschr. Med* 25, 2002, 20.
11 *International Herald Tribune*, 4. 1. 2003.
12 R. Moynihan and R. Smith, 'Too much medicine?', *British Medical Journal* 324, 2002, 859–60.
13 Alexander Dröschel information and quote by personal communication.
14 R. Moynihan, 'Selling sickness: the pharmaceutical industry and disease mongering', *British Medical Journal* 324, 2002, 886–91.
15 K. Dörner, 'In der Fortschrittsfalle', *Deutsches Ärzteblatt* 38, 2002, A-2462.
16 http://www.der-gesunde-mann.de (accessed 22. 4. 2003).
17 Quoted from *Süddeutsche Zeitung*, 14. 1. 2003.
18 H. Füeßl, 'Sagen Sie nicht "Ihnen fehlt nichts"', http://www.mmw.de/wort/indexart.cfm?tree=2&id=1221 (accessed 5. 4. 2003).
19 R. Moynihan, 'Selling sickness: the pharmaceutical industry and disease mongering', *British Medical Journal* 324, 2002, 886–91.
20 All quotes from R. Moynihan, 'Selling sickness: the pharmaceutical industry and disease mongering', *British Medical Journal* 324, 2002, 886–91.

21 Press info of the FDA, 7. 6. 2002 (FDA approves restricted marketing of Lotronex). http://www.pharmavista.ch/indexD.htm?. http://www. pharmavista.ch/news/DVD/00000020D.htm (assessed 6. 1. 2000).

22 J. Cook, 'Practical guide to medical education', *Pharmaceutical Marketing* 6, 2001, 14–22.

23 Figures taken from N. Freemantle and S. Hill, 'Medicalisation, limits to medicine, or never enough money to go around?', *British Medical Journal* 324, 2002, 864–5.

24 Nuffield Council on Bioethics, *Genetics and Human Behaviour: The Ethical Context*, London, 2002. Report online. Available: http://www. nuffieldbioethics.org.

25 According to Gerd Antes from the German Cochrane Zentrum, there are 25,000 medical journals worldwide, which publish every year 2 million research articles.

26 *Ärzte Zeitung*, 14. 5. 2002.

27 R. Porter, *The Greatest Benefit to Mankind*, London, 1997.

28 B. Mintzes, 'Direct to consumer advertising is medicalising normal human experience', *British Medical Journal* 324, 2002, 908–11.

29 E. Taverna, 'Das Dr Knock-Seminar', *Schweizerische Ärztezeitung* 83, 2002, 580.

2 Myths of medicine

1 Press info from the firm Pfizer, 19. 3. 2002.

2 In *Bunte* magazine 27, 2002. See also: http://www.denkpositiv.com

3 C. Ross, 'The informed patient: a step in the right direction'. Online. Available: http://www.Pharmafile.com (accessed 23. 8. 2002).

4 D. Spurgeon, 'Doctors accept $50 a time to listen to drug representatives', *British Medical Journal* 324, 2002, 1113.

5 American physician Bob Goodman looks critically into doctors' susceptibility to corruption: online. Available: http://www.nofreelunch.org.

6 E. Reis et al., 'Qualität und Struktur der ärztlichen Fortbildung in der Inneren Medizin am Beispiel des Ärztekammerbezirks Nordrhein.' *Z. ärztl. Fortbildung. Qual.sich.* 93, 1999, 569–79.

7 N. Choudry et al., 'Relationships between authors of clinical practice guidelines and the pharmaceutical industry', *JAMA* 287, 2002, 612–17.

8 M. Dören, 'Fortbildung in der Sponsoring-Falle?', *Berliner Ärzte* 4, 2003, 18–20.

9 A. Finzen, 'Wir dankbaren Ärzte', *Deutsches Ärzteblatt* 99, 2002, A-766–9.

10 S. Coyle, 'Physician–industry relations. Part 1: Individual physicians', *Annals of Internal Medicine* 136, 2002, 390–402.

11 H. Stelfox, 'Conflict of interest in the debate over calcium-channel antagonists', *New England Journal of Medicine* 338, 1998, p. 101–6.

12 L. Kjaergard, 'Association between competing interests and author's conclusions: epidemiological study of randomised clinical trials published in the BMJ', *British Medical Journal* 325, 2002, 249–52.

13 T. Bodenheimer, 'Uneasy alliance', *New England Journal of Medicine* 342, 2000, 1539–44.

14 FAZ (*Frankfurter Allgemeine Zeitung*), 12. 9. 2001.

15 K. Eichenwald and G. Kolata, 'Drug trials hide conflicts for doctors', *New York Times*, 16. 5. 1999.

16 K. Morin et al., 'Managing conflicts of interest in the conduct of clinical trials', *JAMA* 287, 2002, 78–84.

17 K. Koch, 'Wer rasiert wird, hält besser still', *Süddeutsche Zeitung*, 15. 3. 2002.

18 R. Moynihan, 'The marketing of fear', *Australian Financial Review*, 10. 6. 2000.

19 A. T. Kearney information and quote, press release from German branch.

20 All quotes from R. Moynihan, 'Celebrity selling', *British Medical Journal* 324, 2002, 1342.

21 M. Petersen, 'CNN to reveal when guests promote drugs for companies', *New York Times*, 24. 8. 2002.

22 S. Woloshin et al., 'Direct-to-consumer advertisements for prescription drugs: what are Americans being sold?', *The Lancet* 358, 2001, 1141–6.

23 Referring to the year 1999, quoted from B. Mintzes, 'Direct to consumer advertising is medicalising normal human experience', *British Medical Journal* 324, 2002, 908–9.

24 J. Gammage and K. Stark, 'Under the influence', *Philadelphia Inquirer*, 9. 3. 2002.

25 S. Gottlieb, 'A fifth of Americans contact their doctor as a result of direct to consumer drug advertising', *British Medical Journal* 325, 2002, 854.

26 R. Moynihan et al., 'Coverage by the news media of the benefits and risks of medications', *New England Journal of Medicine* 342, 2000, 1645–50.

3 A disease called diagnosis

1 http://www.osteoporose.org (accessed 22. 11. 2002).

2 K. Müller and S. Müller, *Laborwerte verständlich gemacht*, Stuttgart, 2002.

3 R. Gross, '"Krank" – was ist das eigentlich?', FAZ, 16. 07. 1987.

4 G. Assmann et al., 'Nationale Cholesterin-Initiative', *Deutsches Ärzteblatt* 17 A, 1990, 1358–82.

5 J. Lenzer, 'US consumer body calls for review of cholesterol guidelines', *British Medical Journal* 329, 2004, 759.

6 J. Lenzer, 'Scandals have eroded US public's confidence in drug industry', *British Medical Journal* 329, 2004, 247.

7 Quoted from U. Heyll, *Risikofaktor Medizin*, Frankfurt/Main, 1993.

8 U. Heyll, *Risikofaktor Medizin*, Frankfurt/Main 1993.

9 H. Füeßl, 'Der Check-up macht Patienten froh', *MMW-Fortschr.Med.* 29–30, 2002, 18.

10 J. Blech, 'Bilderwut auf Krankenschein', *Die Zeit* 50, 1996.

11 Sources: *The Orlando Sentinel*, 31. 8. 2002 and *Der Spiegel* 30, 2002.

12 P. Skrabanek and J McCormick, *Follies and Fallacies in Medicine*, Buffalo, CO, 1990.

13 U. Heyll, *Risikofaktor Medizin*, Frankfurt Main, 1993.

14 J. Stone, 'What should we say to patients with symptoms unexplained by disease? The "number needed to offend"', *British Medical Journal* 325, 2002, 1449–50.

15 Quoted freely from P. Skrabanek and J. McCormick, *Follies and Fallacies in Medicine*, Buffalo, CO, 1990.

16 R. Smith, 'In search of "non disease"', British Medical Journal 324, 2002, 883–5.

17 R. Engelhardt, 'Die Moden der Orthopäden', *Die Zeit*, 10. 6. 1999.

18 Source: H. Bakwin, 'Pseudodoxia Pedriatica', *New England Journal of Medicine* 232, 1945, 691.

19 Tamara King, quoted by Jörg Achhammer, 'Wie die Reichen', *Der Tagesspiegel*, 19. 9. 2002, citing *Daily Telegraph*, 18. 9. 2002.

20 D. Gilbert, 'Lifestyle medicines', *British Medical Journal* 321, 2000, 1341–4.

4 The risk factor merry-go-round

1 P. Sawicki, personal statement, April 2003.

2 U. Heyll, *Risikofaktor Medizin*, Frankfurt/Main, 1993.

3 T. Tanne, 'Children should have blood pressure and cholesterol checked by age of 5', *British Medical Journal* 325, 2002, 8.

4 Quoted according to L. Payer, *Disease-Mongers*, New York, 1992.

5 Source: *Der Spiegel* 45, 1990.

6 Paul Rosch, quoted in Uffe Ravnskov with Udo Pollmer, *Mythos Cholesterin*, Stuttgart, 2002, p. 23.

7 *Lancet* quote, in Uffe Ravnskov with Udo Pollmer, *Mythos Cholesterin*, Stuttgart 2002, p. 240.

8 The ten biggest fallacies of the cholesterol theory are described by Uffe Ravnskov with Udo Pollmer in *Mythos Cholesterin*, Stuttgart, 2002. Further information can be found on the Internet: http://www.ravnskov. nu/cholesterol.

9 B. Lown, *Die verlorene Kunst des Heilens*, Stuttgart, 2002.

10 The Heart Protection Study Collaborative Group published its findings in *The Lancet* 360, 7–22: MRC/BHF Heart Protection Study of cholesterol lowering with simvastatin in 20,536 high-risk individuals: a randomised placebo-controlled trial, 2002, 23–33: MRC/BHF Heart Protection Study of antioxidant vitamin supplementation in 20,536 high-risk individuals: a randomised placebo-controlled trial, 2002.

11 K. Koch, 'Ein Volk von Kranken', *Süddeutsche Zeitung*, 8. 2. 2002.

12 For example: Bayer, Aventis, MerckSharpDome, Novartis, Sanofi-Synthelabo, Hoffmann-La Roche, AstraZeneca, Medisana, Omron Medizintechnik, Bristol-Myers Squibb or Pfizer. See http://www.paritaet.org/ hochdruckliga/welcome.htm.

13 R. Bretzel, 'Diabetes und Insulin', *Druckpunkt* 3, 2002, 8.

14 P. Little, 'Comparison of agreement between different measures of blood pressure in primary care and daytime ambulatory blood pressure', *British Medical Journal* 325, 2002, 254–7.

15 U. Heyll, *Risikofaktor Medizin*, Frankfurt/Main, 1993.

16 Quoted according to C. Green, 'Bone mineral density testing: does the evidence support its selective use in well women?', *Vancouver, BC: British Columbia Office of Health Technology Assessment*, 1997.

17 An identical definition for osteoporosis can be found, for example, in a WHO memo from April 1999: http://www.who.int/archives/whday/en/documents1999/osteo.html.

18 Quotation from *Der Spiegel* 14, 1998.

19 Quoted from *Osteoporose aktuell 2002*, a brochure of the Federal Self-Help-Association for Osteoporosis.

20 G. Gawlik, 'Entscheidung über umstrittene Methoden', *Deutsches Ärzteblatt* 97, 2000, A-819.

21 C. Green, 'Bone mineral density testing; does the evidence support its selective use in well women?', *Vancouver, BC: British Columbia Office of Health Technology Assessment*, 1997.

22 *MMW-Fortschr. Med* 5, 2003.

23 The list of risk factors is growing longer each day; this one is taken from P. Skrabanek and J. McCormick, *Follies and Fallacies in Medicine*, Buffalo, CO, 1990.

24 The quotations are by G. S. Myers and Dr Howard, taken from P. Skrabanek and J. McCormick, *Follies and Fallacies in Medicine*, Buffalo, CO, 1990.

5 Insanity as the norm

1 R. Schneider, 'Acht flogen über das Kuckucksnest', *Neue Züricher Zeitung*, 2. 9. 2002.

2 D. Rosenhan, 'On being sane in insane places', *Science* 179, 1973, 250–8.

3 Press info from the German Society for Psychiatry, Psychotherapy and Mental Health, September 2002.

4 D. Healy, *The Creation of Psychopharmacology*, Cambridge, MA and London, 2002.

5 Eli Lilly letter: 'Controversial disease dropped from Prozac product information', *British Medical Journal* 328, 2004, 365.

6 A. Finzen and U. Hoffmann-Richter, 'Schöne neue Diagnosenwelt', *Soziale Psychiatrie* 1, 2002.

7 J. Brown, 'The next wave of psychotherapeutic drugs: a new generation of drugs are in development to tackle a wide range of mental illnesses', *Med Ad News* 21, 2002, 38.

8 A. Huxley, *Brave New World*, 1932.

9 *The New York Times*, 30. 6. 2002, quote by A. A. Levin, director of the Center of Medical Consumers.

10 Press info from the German Society for Psychiatry, Psychotherapy and Mental Health, June 2001.

11 Connection between SmithKline Beecham and coalition: 'First, you market the disease . . . then you push the pills to treat it: Brendan I Kocrncr on the ugly truth about doctors, PR firms and drug companies', *Guardian*, 30. 7. 2002.

12 M. Cottle, 'Diagnose Menschenscheu', *Neue Züricher Zeitung*, 18. 3. 2000.

13 Quoted according to B. Koerner, 'First you market the disease . . . then you push the pills to treat it', *Guardian*, 30. 7. 2002.

14 Jack Gorman quoted in *Guardian*: 'First, you market the disease . . . then you push the pills to treat it: Brendan I Koerner on the ugly truth about doctors, PR firms and drug companies', *Guardian*, 30. 7. 2002.

15 Source: *Die Zeit*, 15. 11. 2001.
16 A. Finzen, *Warum werden unsere Kranken eigentlich wieder gesund?*, Bonn, 2002.

6 Psycho pill with break-time snack

1 Quoted from J. Blech and K. Thimm, 'Kinder mit Knacks', *Der Spiegel* 29, 2002.
2 Press info from the German Society for Psychiatry, Psychotherapy and Mental Health, November 2002.
3 Novartis brochure, undated.
4 J. Brown, 'The next wave of psychotherapeutic drugs: a new generation of drugs are in development to tackle a wide range of mental illnesses', *Med Ad News* 21, 2002, 38.
5 Quoted according to J. Swanson, 'Attention-deficit hyperactivity disorder and hyperkinetic disorder', *The Lancet* 351, 1998, 429–33.
6 Ciba-Geigy merged with Sandoz in 1996 to form Novartis, the present-day producer of Ritalin.
7 P. Schrag and D. Divoky, *The Myth of the Hyperactive Child*, New York, 1975.
8 P. Schrag and D. Divoky, *The Myth of the Hyperactive Child*, New York, 1975.
9 The supplement brochure of the journal *Kinder- und Jugendarzt* 1, 2002, was published under the title 'Be quiet – don't dream – pay attention!'
10 Source: programme of the symposium that took place on 19. 10. 2002 in Stade.
11 Clipping from *Ärztliche Praxis* paper.
12 Skrodski information, researched by Jörg Blech. Printed in *Der Spiegel* 29, 2002.
13 Press bulletin of the German Society for Psychiatry, Psychotherapy and Mental Health, March 2002; according to the imprint this 'Press info psychiatry and psychotherapy' was published with the support of the companies Astra Zeneca, Aventis Pharmaceutical Deutschland GmbH, Lilly, Novartis Pharmaceutical and Organon.
14 J. Smoller, 'The etiology and treatment of childhood', *Journal of Polymorphous Perversity* 2, 1985, 3–7.
15 Quoted from J. Blech and K. Thimm, 'Kinder mit Knacks', *Der Spiegel* 29, 2002.
16 Source: *Der Spiegel* 29, 2002.
17 Source: *Der Spiegel* 29, 2002.
18 S. Stolberg, 'Preschool Meds', *New York Times Magazine*, 17. 11. 2002.
19 J. Swanson, 'Attention-deficit hyperactivity disorder and hyperkinetic disorder', *The Lancet* 351, 1998, 429–33.
20 H. Hafer, *Die heimliche Droge: Nahrungsphosphat*, Karl F. Haug Verlag, Heidelberg, 1997.
21 R. Barkley, 'Hyperaktive Kinder', *Spektrum der Wissenschaft* 8, 2000.
22 Special issue 'Unaufmerksam und hyperaktiv' of *Kinderärztliche Praxis*, 15. 1. 2001.

23 N. Volkow, 'Therapeutic doses of oral methylphenidate significantly increase extracellular dopamine in the human brain', *Journal of Neuroscience* 21, 2001, RC121 (1–5).
24 J. Elia et al., 'Treatment of attention-deficit-hyperactivity disorder', *New England Journal of Medicine* 340, 1999, 780–7.
25 G. Moll, 'Early methylphenidate administration to young rats causes a persistent reduction in the density of striatal dopamine transporters', *Journal of Child and Adolescent Psychopharmacology* 11, 2001, 15–24.
26 G. Hüther, 'Kritische Anmerkungen zu den bei ADHD-Kindern beobachteten neurobiologischen Veränderungen und den vermuteten Wirkungen von Psychostimulanzien (Ritalin)', *Analytische Kinder- und Jugendlichen-Psychotherapie* 112, 2001, 471.
27 K. Brown, 'The medication merry-go-round', *Science* 299, 2003, 1646–9.
28 F. Fukuyama, 'Life, but not as we know it', *New Scientist* 20. 4. 2002.
29 Source: *Geo* 3, 2003.

7 The femininity syndrome

1 Quoted from E. Shorter, *Moderne Leiden*, Reinbeck bei Hamburg, 1994.
2 Quoted from E. Shorter, *Moderne Leiden*, Reinbeck bei Hamburg, 1994.
3 P. Kolip (ed.), *Weiblichkeit ist keine Krankheit*, Weinheim and Munich, 2000.
4 J. Aronson, 'When I use a word . . . medicalisation', *British Medical Journal* 324, 2002, 904.
5 Source: *Women's Health*, no date or issue number mentioned, taken from a gynaecological practice in Hamburg in September 2002.
6 Schindele information from P. Kolip (ed.), *Weiblichkeit ist keine Krankheit*, Weinheim and Munich, 2000.
7 Quoted from P. Kolip (ed.), *Weiblichkeit ist keine Krankheit*, Weinheim and Munich, 2000.
8 Quoted from K. Müller's contribution 'Die Entfernung der "nutzlosen" Gebärmutter', in P. Kolip (ed.), *Weiblichkeit ist keine Krankheit*, Weinheim and Munich, 2000.
9 J. Schaffer and A. Word, 'Hysterectomy – still a useful operation', *New England Journal of Medicine* 347, 2002, 1360–2.
10 In France, 90 out of 100,000 women per year have a hysterectomy and in Germany 357 out of 100,000 per year. Figures according to Kolip 2000.
11 S. Wagner, 'Wenn die "rote" Tante zu Besuch ist', *Weltwoche*, 8. 3. 2001.
12 S. Westphal, 'Lifting the curse', *New Scientist*, 16. 3. 2002.
13 A. Tsao, 'Freedom from the menstrual cycle?', *Business Week online*, 23. 5. 2003.
14 A. Tsao, 'Freedom from the menstrual cycle?', *Business Week online*, 23. 5. 2003.
15 S. Westphal, 'Lifting the curse', *New Scientist*, 16. 3. 2002.
16 Quoted from P. Kolip (ed.), *Weiblichkeit ist keine Krankheit*, Weinheim and Munich, 2000.
17 This is the result of a survey among 8,440 women; it was presented in May 2002 at the conference of the German Society for Obstetrics in Hamburg.
18 *taz*, 9. 11. 2001

19 All quotations from R. Essig, 'Geburt mit Wein und Dolch', *Die Zeit* 52, 2002, 43.

20 A. Zaremba, 'The new Latin labour', *Nunnamuid*, P.G. 9. 2001.

21 R. Johanson, 'Has the medicalisation of childbirth gone too far?', *British Medical Journal* 324, 2002, 892–5.

22 Press info from the German Society for Psychiatry, Psychotherapy and Mental Health from April 2001.

23 P. Husslein, 'Frauen müssen wählen dürfen', *Medical Tribune* 41, 2002, 14.

24 M. Wagner, 'Choosing Caesarean Section', *The Lancet* 356, 2000, 1677–80.

25 *Ärzte Zeitung*, 22. 5. 2002.

26 E.-J. Hickl and H. Franzki, 'Indikationen zur Sectio caesarea – Zur Frage der sog. Sectio auf Wunsch', *Der Gynäkologe* 2, 2002, 197–202.

27 R. A. Wilson, *Feminine Forever*, M. Evans and Lippincott, New York, 1966.

28 G. Kolata with M. Petersen, 'Hormone replacement study: a shock to the medical system', *New York Times*, 10. 7. 2002.

29 B. Wanner, 'Menopause: Im Spannungsfeld der Paradigmen', *Neue Zürcher Zeitung*, 28. 1. 1998.

30 *Deutsches Ärzteblatt* 97, 2000, A-2512–6.

31 D. Elschenbroich, 'Wie es ist, ist es gut', *Frankfurter Allgemeine Zeitung*, 28. 6. 1995.

32 B. Wanner, 'Menopause: Im Spannungsfeld der Paradigmen', *Neue Zürcher Zeitung*, 28. 1. 1998.

33 All quotations from *Der Spiegel* 43, 1991.

34 Source: *Neue Zürcher Zeitung am Sonntag*, 28. 4. 2002.

35 Quoted from K. Koch, 'Auf der Suche nach der Wahrheit', *Süddeutsche Zeitung*, 20. 3. 2001.

36 Quoted from *Süddeutsche Zeitung*, 17. 9. 2002.

37 D. Grady et al., 'Cardiovascular disease outcomes during 6.8 years of hormone therapy', *JAMA* 288, 2002, 49–57.

38 Writing group for the women's health initiative investigators, 'Risks and benefits of oestrogen plus progestin in healthy postmenopausal women', *JAMA* 288, 2002, 321–33.

39 Information about Jenopharm fax claim: Hormonersatztherapie: Aufklärung mit freundlicher Unterstützung, Deutsches Ärzteblatt 99, Ausgabe 31–32 vom 05.08.2002, Seite A-2088/B-1768/C-1664.

40 J. Hays, 'Effects of oestrogen plus progestin on health-related quality of life', *New England Journal of Medicine*. Online. Available: http://www.nejm.org (accessed 17 March 2003).

41 In a press release dated 3. 9. 2002.

42 The *arznei-telegramm* informs critically and independently about medicinal drugs and therapies; quotation is taken from *arznei-telegramm* 8, 2002. See also http://www.arznei-telegramm.de.

8 Old men, new afflictions

1 Press release from Schuster Public Relations & Media Consulting, 30. 10. 2002.

2 Brochure *Fragen und Antworten* of the firms Dr Kade/Besins and Solvay Arzneimittel, not dated.
3 R. Kirby (ed.), *Männerheilkunde*, Bern, 2002.
4 Brochure *Fragen und Antworten* of the firms Dr Kade/Besins and Solvay Arzneimittel, not dated.
5 Brochure *Fragen und Antworten* of the firms Dr Kade/Besins and Solvay Arzneimittel, not dated.
6 Press info from the firm Jenapharm, March 2003.
7 'Report of National Institute on Aging Advisory Panel on Testosterone Replacement in Men', *Journal of Clinical Endocrinology and Metabolism* 86 (10), 2001, 4611–14.
8 Consensus Paper 'Der alternde Mann', *Reproduktionsmedizin* 16, 2000, 439–40.
9 J. Groopman, 'Hormones for men', *New Yorker* 31, 2002.
10 S. von Eckardstein and E. Nieschlag, 'Therapie mit Sexualhormonen beim alternden Mann', *Deutsches Ärzteblatt* 97, A-3175–82, 2000.
11 J. Blech, 'Neue Leiden alter Männer', *Der Spiegel* 16, 2003.
12 Press info from the firm Jenapharm, December 2002.
13 J. Groopman, 'Hormones for men', *New Yorker* 31, 2002.
14 'Report of National Institute on Aging Advisory Panel on Testosterone Replacement in Men', *Journal of Clinical Endocrinology and Metabolism* 86 (10), 2001, 4611–14.
15 A. Morales and B. Lunenfeld, 'Androgen replacement therapy in aging men with secondary hypogonadism', *The Aging Male* 4, 2001, 151–62.
16 P. Snyder, 'Effect of testosterone treatment on bone mineral density in men over 65 years of age', *Journal of Clinical Endocrinology and Metabolism* 84, 1999, 1966–72.
17 Source: *Abrechnungsleitfaden für den Arzt*, from Dr Kade/Besins and Solvay Arzneimittel, not dated.
18 G. Stockinger, 'Viagra für den ganzen Körper', *Der Spiegel* 29, 2000.
19 G. Kolata, 'Testosterone use prompts concern among doctors', *New York Times*, 22. 08. 2002.
20 A. Brown and N. Comer-Calder, 'The unstoppable power of the male menopause', *Observer*, 24. 03. 2002.
21 I. Owens, 'Sex differences in mortality rate', *Science* 297, 2002, 2008–9.
22 S. Moore and K. Wilson, 'Parasites as a viability cost of sexual selection in natural populations of mammals', *Science* 297, 2002, 2015–18.
23 J. Olshansky, 'No truth to the fountain of youth', *Scientific American* 6, 2002.
24 Ibid.
25 Source: *Der Spiegel* 21, 2002.

9 Whenever you want it

1 W. Schultz et al., 'Magnetic resonance imaging of male and female genitals during coitus and female sexual arousal', *British Medical Journal* 319, 1999, 1596–600.
2 J. Blech, 'Die zweite sexuelle Revolution', *Der Spiegel* 7, 2002.
3 J. Hitt, 'The second sexual revolution', *New York Times Magazine*, 20. 2. 2000.

4 G. Hart and K. Wellings, 'Sexual behaviour and its medicalisation: in sickness and in health', *British Medical Journal* 324, 2002, 896–900.
5 Quoted from *Observer*, 11. 02. 2001.
6 R. Moynihan, 'The making of a disease. female sexual dysfunction', *British Medical Journal* 326, 2003, 45–7.
7 R. Moynihan, 'The making of a disease: female sexual dysfunction', *British Medical Journal* 326, 2003, 45–7.
8 E. Laumann et al., 'Sexual dysfunction in the United States: prevalence and predictors', *JAMA* 281, 1999, 537–44.
9 J. Kaye and J. Hershel, 'Incidence of erectile dysfunction and characteristics of patients before and after the introduction of sildenafil in the United Kingdom: cross-sectional study with comparison patients', *British Medical Journal* 326, 2003, 424–5.
10 G. Hart and K. Wellings, 'Sexual behaviour and its medicalisation: in sickness and in health', *British Medical Journal* 324, 2002, 896–900.
11 http://www.lilly-pharma.de (accessed 1 March 2003).
12 http://www.der-gesunde-mann.de (accessed 1 March 2003).
13 All figures according to J. P. Pryor, 'Editorial', *BJU International* 88, 2001, 3.
14 M. Petersen, 'Advertising – Pfizer, facing competition from other drug makers, looks for a younger market for Viagra', *New York Times*, 13. 2. 2002.
15 R. Moynihan, 'Urologist recommends daily Viagra to prevent impotence', *British Medical Journal* 326, 2003, 9.
16 Quoted from *Observer*, 11. 2. 2001. Leonore Tiefer has organised a campaign against female sexual dysfunction, see http://www.fsd-alert.org

10 Destiny in our genes

1 Internet sites of the companies can be found at http://www.gentest24.de and www.gen-untersuchung.com (Zentrum für Individuelle Diagnostik). See as well: H. Berth, 'Entwicklung mit Risiken', *Deutsches Ärzteblatt* 40, 2002, A-2599–2603.
2 Quoted from *Guardian*, 4. 6. 2002.
3 U. Wiesing (ed.), *Ethik in der Medizin*, Stuttgart, 2000.
4 A regularly updated list of available gene tests can be found on the Internet at http://www.geneclinics.org
5 G. Feuerstein and R. Kollek, 'Vom genetischen Wissen zum sozialen Risiko: Gendiagnostik als Instrument der Biopolitik', *Das Parlament* 27, 2001. Online. Available: http://www.das-parlament.de/2001/27/Beilage/2001 27 005 5834.html
6 D. Galton and G. Ferns, 'Genetic markers to predict polygenic disease: a new problem for social genetics', *Quarterly Journal of Medicine* 92, 2002, 223–32.
7 W. Burke, 'Genetic Testing', *New England Journal of Medicine* 347, 2002, 1867–75.
8 D. Melzer and R. Zimmern, 'Genetics and medicalisation', *British Medical Journal* 324, 2002, 863–4.
9 L. Temple et al., 'Defining diseases in the genomics era', *Science* 293, 2001, 807–8.

150 *Notes*

10 D. Melzer and R. Zimmern, 'Genetics and medicalisation', *British Medical Journal* 324, 2002, 863–4.
11 D. Galton and G. Ferns, 'Genetic markers to predict polygenic disease: a new problem for social genetics', *Quarterly Journal of Medicine* 92, 2002, 223–32.
12 W. Burke, 'Genetic testing', *New England Journal of Medicine* 347, 2002, 1867–75.
13 D. Galton and G. Ferns, 'Genetic markers to predict polygenic disease: a new problem for social genetics', *Quarterly Journal of Medicine* 92, 2002, 223–32.
14 D. Josefson, 'Doctors successfully screen embryos for gene mutation linked to early onset of Alzheimer's', *British Medical Journal* 324, 2002, 564.
15 *Der Spiegel* 41, 2000.

11 Healthy beyond belief

1 L. Payer, *Disease-Mongers*, New York, 1992.
2 U. Popert, 'Ouvertüre oder Abgesang?', *Deutsches Ärzteblatt* 6, 2003, A-302.
3 Reader's letter in *MMW-Fortschritte der Medizin* 46, 2002, 18.
4 A. Sen, 'Health perception versus observation', *British Medical Journal* 324, 2002, 860–1.
5 Information from 2002; see also http://www.who.int/medicines.
6 R. Böger, 'Wie wird die chronische Herzinsuffizienz heute tatsächlich behandelt?', *Deutsche Medizinische Wochenschrift* 127, 2002, 1764–8.
7 *MMW-Fortschritte der Medizin* 25, 2002.
8 E. Gerharz, 'Größenwahn? Die psychosozialen Konsequenzen von Kleinwuchs', *Deutsches Ärzteblatt* 14, 2003, A925–8.
9 *The Economist*, 25. 5. 2002.
10 W. Harth, 'Lifestyle-Medikamente und körperdysmorphe Störungen', *Deutsches Ärzteblatt* 3, 2003, A 128–31.
11 J. Le Fanu, *The Rise and Fall of Modern Medicine*, New York, 2000.
12 J. Blech, 'Arme sterben früher', *Die Zeit* 43, 1997.
13 G. Kaiser, *Die Zukunft der Medizin*, Frankfurt/Main, 1996.
14 J. Savulescu and J. Kerin, 'The "geneticisation" of disease stigma', *Lancet* 354, 1999, 16.
15 J. Blech, 'Das Ende', *Die Zeit* 30, 1997.
16 I. Illich, *Die Nemesis der Medizin*, fourth revised edn, Munich, 1995.
17 R. Moynihan and R. Smith, 'Too much medicine?', *British Medical Journal* 324, 2002, 859–60.
18 D. Gilbert et al., 'Lifestyle medicines', *British Medical Journal* 321, 2000, 1341–4.
19 Nuffield Council on Bioethics, *Genetics and Human Behaviour: The Ethical Context*, London, 2002. Online. Available: http://www.nuffield-bioethics.org
20 *Spiegel* 19, 2002.
21 Source: Reader's letter in *Deutsches Ärzteblatt* 16, a-1081.
22 H. Raspe, 'Ethische Implikationen der Evidenz-basierten Medizin', *Deutsche Medizinische Wochenschrift* 127, 2002, 1769–73.

23 Quoted according to K. Bergdolt, *Leib und Seele*, Munich, 1999.
24 B. Lown, *Die verlorene Kunst des Heilens*, Stuttgart, 2002.
25 P. Skrabanek and J. McCormick, *Follies and Fallacies in Medicine*, Buffalo, NY, 1990.

Internet addresses

General

Information comprehensible to the medical laity on selected diseases as well as examination and treatment methods offered by the University of Witten/Herdecke http://www.patientenleitlinien.de; primarily for physicians http://www.evidence.de

Generally comprehensible science-based statements on medicine, hygiene and health care by experts in the field of health from the University of Hamburg http://www.gesundheit.uni-hamburg.de

The *arznei-telegramm* informs critically and independently about drugs and therapies http://www.arznei-telegramm.de

Databases

Medline (Pubmed) http://www.ncbi.nlm.nih.gov
DIMDI: German Institute for Medical Documentation and Information http://www.dimdi.de/dynamic/en/index.html

Search engines

TRIP database http://www.tripdatabase.com/index.cfm
Sum search http://sumsearch.uthscsa.edu/searchform45.htm

Evidence-based medicine

DIeM Institut für evidenzbasierte Medizin in Cologne
http://www.di-em.de
German Network for Evidence Based Medicine
http://www.ebm-netzwerk.de/english
Deutsches Cochrane Zentrum http://www.cochrane.de

Ulmer Initiative für Evidence-based Medicine
http://www.uni-ulm.de/cebm/
NHS Centre for Reviews and Dissemination, University of York
http://www.york.ac.uk/inst/crd/
Cochrane Collaboration Consumer Network
http://www.cochraneconsumer.com

Medical journals

http://<www.freemedicaljournals.com
British Medical Journal http://www.bmj.com
Journal of the American Medical Association http://www.jama.com
EBM-Online http://ebm.bmjjournals.com

Information on medicinal drugs

Bundesinstitut für Arzneimittel und Medizinprodukte
http://www.bfarm.de
European Agency for the Evaluation of Medical Products
http://www.emea.eu.int
Food and Drug Administration http://www.fda.gov

Index

Printed in the United States
by Baker & Taylor Publisher Services